CAZ HOW

The Social Substance

Understanding the Lie that is Alcohol

First published by CazHow Productions 2023

Copyright © 2023 by Caz How

All rights reserved. No part of this publication may be reproduced, stored or transmitted in any form or by any means, electronic, mechanical, photocopying, recording, scanning, or otherwise without written permission from the publisher. It is illegal to copy this book, post it to a website, or distribute it by any other means without permission.

Caz How asserts the moral right to be identified as the author of this work.

Caz How has no responsibility for the persistence or accuracy of URLs for external or third-party Internet Websites referred to in this publication and does not guarantee that any content on such Websites is, or will remain, accurate or appropriate.

Designations used by companies to distinguish their products are often claimed as trademarks. All brand names and product names used in this book and on its cover are trade names, service marks, trademarks and registered trademarks of their respective owners. The publishers and the book are not associated with any product or vendor mentioned in this book. None of the companies referenced within the book have endorsed the book.

Caz How does not profess to be a medical 'expert' regarding any content in this book. Any advice and opinions given herein are qualified solely by the author's own life experiences.

First edition

ISBN: 978-0-6459615-1-5

Cover art by Lara Amro

This book was professionally typeset on Reedsy. Find out more at reedsy.com

For my fellow drinkers...

*The carnival is over
The lights have dimmed down low
But a new world has arisen
in a heavenly sober glow*

*I invite you on this journey
I promise you such light
on the other side of drinking
Where your New Life is in sight.*

Contents

Preface		ii
Acknowledgement		iv
1	Introduction	1
2	Meet Me At The Local	5
3	The Downward Spiral	12
4	The Final Drinking Years	23
5	The Fucking Lie That Is Alcohol	33
6	Drinking and Dating	48
7	Drinking and Parenting	57
8	Uncategorised Chaos	63
9	How Do I Stop?	71
10	But Can I Moderate (Or Not)?	91
11	The Decision	106
12	It's More Fun Not Drinking!	123
13	Q & A Time!	134
14	Conclusion	147
Afterword		148
About the Author		149

Preface

This book came about in a somewhat unusual way.

At the time of writing it, or more accurately, commencing the Punchy Book writing course which culminated in my finishing a manuscript for a change, I was around three and a half years sober. And I'd been writing since I was in high school, where my English teacher suggested to me I'd be a writer one day. My attitude being such that it was, I scoffed at the suggestion, and embarked upon a lifetime of drinking instead!

I've worked with words for most of my life - always typing other people's words, for money. I've privately typed plenty of my own, but these have never seen the light of day - till now. Some might argue it's best they remain hidden - but you be the judge.

This book really materialised, though, when I scored a new gig, doing live media captioning. The job entailed respeaking other people's words - yes, here I was again, working with *other people's words* - but most intolerable for me, having to respeak them verbatim, even if the words were blatant lies. You know, things like red wine is good for you.. or a slab of beer a day leads to a more exciting sex life... or governments are comprised of kind, altruistic, selfless folk.

The salary was great. But the moral cost was too high - frankly unbearable.

So I downed tools – and began a writing course – and then wrote this book. All my words, my design, for better or worse, and all at the tender age of 59 years young at time of publishing.

But I know I could never have completed a mission like this as a drinker.

This is my story, in all its good, bad, funny, and downright sticky bits. Real, embarrassing, and yet full of hope, and seriously radical joy!

Caz How – September 2023

Acknowledgement

It's here I need to thank all of those who've come - and gone - and in some instances, stayed - in my life over the decades, because each one of you has contributed to my shift in awareness, and then wanting, and finally achieving my joyful, sober life purpose.

I'm sorry I took so long - but I got here eventually.

Thank you, with heartfelt gratitude. You know who you are.

1

Introduction

Do you ever wonder about your own relationship with alcohol, as opposed to that of others around you, like family and friends?

Have you checked out those online quizzes – 'Are you an alcoholic?' – or even privately filled one out – for a friend, of course...

Does it baffle you that you *know* you want to control your drinking - yet seem to do the exact opposite?

Have you always accepted that your friends are being honest regarding their alcohol usage, or do you question if they too might be hiding what's believed to be this 'shameful and private' problem?

Do you feel alone in your lack of control around the social substance?

Have your relationships suffered, with problems put on the back burner, because of regular alcohol use?

Are you unable to make decisions, or positive change, because you feel too tired? Or are you waking each morning in a joyless state?

Perhaps you've secretly dreamed of checking into a rehab centre for a rest, where the problem is blissfully taken away from you, and you get to emerge after 90 days as a happy undrinker? (if only it weren't so expensive, and ultimately ineffective in the long term).

I'm here to debunk a lot of myths around alcohol.

Because particularly here in Australia, where we have ads on the TV that implore us, first and foremost, to *Save the XXXX beer!* - it's clear that our cultural mindset is drinking at all costs. And if it's to excess, whether once, or occasionally, or most times, well, that's just part of the fun!

But when it's not fun anymore, well, it's now *your* problem!

Your lack of control.

You, my friend, are an undisciplined piss-head, separated from the *masses* who manage to drink daily, socially, or occasionally, all without problem.

Just YOU.

So best you keep *your* problem to *yourself.*

But - keep drinking and 'having fun', for fuck's sake!

I'm going to take you through a journey of understanding regarding our social substance.

It's not what the man at the bottle-o will tell you, or the government-endorsed labels on their products fall short of, or the adverts for gambling, or a social day at the races will confirm for you.

It's not even what an alcohol counsellor might spruik – because I'm going to suggest their best financial interests (obviously) lie in your ongoing problem, not in the solution.

INTRODUCTION

Over my roughly four decades of love/hate drinking, I can tell you I tried everything to get the beast under control (just so I could continue drinking, of course!)

I did Ocsobers, Dry Julys. Movembers (that one failed, because my moustache grew back). I desperately moderated. I even abstained totally - until I couldn't. I did willpower to death. I stoically trudged the 12 Steps. I attended counselling. I read numerous books, including one or two good ones, on the topic.

I spoke to friends and strangers. And my friends mostly insisted I didn't have a problem!

Go figure.

Mine is a personal journey of enlightenment on the fraud that is alcohol, of its dangers, and its readiness to destroy lives – and not just mine.

I learnt that turning to the bottle solves nothing; it just put off the day when I could make positive changes in my life.

This is a journey of understanding that the buck really stopped with me – and always had – for nigh on 40 years. That there's no such thing as infinite willpower – because that runs out regularly – so I needed something *within* to turn to when the going got rocky. And I needed to practise that skill, every day, because initially, like learning anything new, it takes work. Until it becomes automatic – and finally, blissfully, it's beautiful, fresh subconscious wiring. With a spritz of lime!

Blaming others, or situations, or life's problems for your drinking takes the responsibility and power away from you to improve your own life.

Also, there's no counsellor on earth that can stop you drinking when you want to, or when those conditions line up for your next drink. No hypnotist, no faith healer, no 12-step program, no rehab revolving door – nothing but yourself.

It's your own understanding of what's *really* at play here, and your willingness to look at the problem in a whole new way, with your own unique solution. It's a true reality check on what this socially-endorsed substance really is, and what it does to your brain over time.Why you're more valuable to the economy hooked, than sober.

And from there, you'll realise that until you truly understand and ingest the truth about alcohol, you'll never really be free of it.Because it's all around you, just waiting for your next bad day, to invite it back in.

Are you ready to explore it a different way?

I invite you to join me. We're going to time-travel back to my drinking days, just this once – so we can talk about it over a beer. Yep, in that bar down the road.

2

Meet Me At The Local

Scene – the local Bowls Club

Once upon a time, I was waking up every Saturday morning hungover and depressed.

Sometimes Sunday mornings too.

And then weekday mornings.

And as much as I agonized that I just couldn't go on like this – somehow – I did.

So, I normalized it by believing *hell, everyone drinks, so it must be okay*. And I lost hope of ever climbing out of the trap.

At that stage, I firmly believed that *not* drinking wasn't an option for me. Because I'd seen those types - you know the ones. They'd be hanging around at a party, clutching a glass of soda water that they'd tried to make look exciting by having it in a tall glass with ice and a wedge of lime – but they weren't fooling *me* – or themselves.

I knew they weren't having any fun, *couldn't* be having any fun. What they were was delusional!

Oops hang on a second, I just spilt my beer 'cos some drunken dickhead crashed into me on his way back from the bar. What a waste of good beer.

Anyway, where was I?

Oh, that's right, I was talking about that sad loser over there, still clutching his un-spilt soda, and pretending he's having a good time without alcohol.

You don't fool me, buddy.

I've done Ocsober, and I know what it's like.

In fact, you're pissing me off even *being* at a venue like this, pretending you can enjoy yourself. You're like a leashed dog on a leash-free dog beach. Frustrated.

And I might go over there and set you straight. But I better go replenish my refreshment first, I haven't had quite enough yet to be in my best form.

Hang about.

#

Sorry that took so long – the bar was ten deep. And I ran into some friends there.

I always do, at this place. It's great to see them, to be the life of the party again. They always show me they're happy to see me too, although sometimes it's in ways I don't like. Like that creepy guy who always gets his thrills by pinching me on the rear to attract my attention, in the hope I might then turn around for him to eyeball my tits.

Ah well, he's only human. And he won't care that I smell like a brewery now. My boozy waft is his Chanel No.5.

Make it a pint this time – it'll save me lining up again so soon. I'd buy two at a time, but then I have to drink it faster so it doesn't warm up.

If only someone would invent a way to keep beer colder for longer, or something really useful like that. Yeah, just make it a pint.

Okay, so listen up.

Alcohol makes you feel the way you ought to be able to feel without alcohol!

And that is my pearl of wisdom, my friends.

Well, not the only one.

But it's why I drink.

It's why, I suspect, many of us drink. And that's why it's weird when people don't drink.

I can't work it out.

I mean, do they really feel like they're *actually enough* without it? Oh, no way. Look at them. They don't look enough to me.

I mean, I will talk to non-drinkers, of course. I don't *enjoy* it, but hey, I'm a charitable kind of gal. With beer in hand, I can literally talk to a stone statue and make it laugh back. But talking to non-drinkers – meh. They're just boring, right. Mournful, even. And I don't want to be around mournful.

That's why I drink…

(Shocked eyes, peering into myself at this point).

Is that why I drink? Really? Who said that?

I thought the real reason I drank is because it alleviates my stress?

(I take another look).

Okay, no one else is listening here, so I'll tell you a little story about that.

Move in closer.

This is just for you.

#

A while back, I saw this book called 'The Alcohol Experiment' in my local bookstore. And of course, I flicked through it. Idly – of course – I was just killing time.

I mean, I don't have a problem with drinking, but I can understand that some people do. That's why AA exists.

But anyway, I picked up this book, and it kind of *lured* me in. The chapters were short. And besides, I like experiments, they're so – er – experimental, and exciting.

So, one of the first things this book informed me I should do, was to make a list. The list had to contain the reasons why I drank – or why I thought I drank. And having done that, I then had to make a second list, and this would contain the reasons why I no longer *wanted* to drink.

Fascinating. I put the book down, and walked out, with lists rapidly forming in my thoughts. And because I'm a quasi-writer (but never had time to finish a book, too busy drinking – oops – enjoying life!) I went home and actually committed pencil to paper. And I came up with a stack of reasons for my first list, and alleviating my stress came out tops.

Second on that list was that the booze was essential to relax me for social events, because being an event organizer, I needed that mojo to keep the punters returning for more fun. There was a stack of other reasons, all legitimate of course, which I now can't quite remember.

And then I got to the second list. Reasons why I no longer wanted to drink.

Hmmm.

Well, I *did* want to keep drinking.

(Didn't I?)

I glanced down in horror as my pencil seemed to grow legs, and began scribbling bullet points into that second list, which sat on a facing pace to my first list. And I watched in lurid fascination as not just one or two points appeared, but then kept on spilling out, like vomit onto the page.

Pretty soon, I'd outstripped that first list, and was *still* going. It was incredible. Here I had come up with about ten reasons why I drank, and about double why I no longer wanted to!

I dropped the pencil, furrowed my brow in what I hoped was an intelligent, enlightened manner, and allowed the first couple of contradictions to marinate in my shocked brain.

I drink alcohol to alleviate stress

But:

I want to stop drinking because my behavior stresses me out.

And then:

I drink alcohol because it relaxes me as an organizer, and makes people like me.

But:

I don't want to drink because I act like a dick around people socially, get rude and obnoxious, and I'm becoming known as a piss-head.

I realised I'd chewed the end off my pencil. My teeth hurt. And so did my brain.

What the fuck was going on here?

#

So, that was the beginning for me. And although I didn't buy that book that day, I did eventually, a long time later, when I knew that it was the start of my realising something:

The Lie That Is Alcohol.

The realisations just kept on spilling out of me, after that point.

I couldn't stop them.

Anytime I got sober (usually on a weekday) I would feel kind of down. Kind of like I was just waiting to have fun again.

My life went on hold while I wasn't drinking. I just carried on with this drudgery called Life, while I waited for *"it's five o'clock somewhere in the world"* to rock around again.

I longed for the time I could crack open those beers, so I could then have some fun.

Because there was no fun to be had without it.

There was no fun with it either, is how I always felt afterwards though – till the next time.

Problem – reaction – solution.

Keep drinking.

I need it because I feel stressed about stuff I can't change.

But I feel stressed about the stupid shit I do when I'm on the drink.

I feel stressed about what I'm doing to my brain, my body, my health.

I love myself when I drink, because people love me when I drink. I'm so much fun, they tell me!

But I hate myself the next day. I'm embarrassed about what I might have done, because I can't even remember what I did. Who did I offend? Who did I ignore?

Oh – and where the fuck is my phone; did I lose it yet again last night?

Wait – that last one falls under the stress category, you goose. Pay attention.

At this point, I was beginning to realise something pretty massive, and it had to do with The Lie That Is Alcohol.

The Contradiction that is Alcohol.

That the shit wasn't serving me anymore, if it ever had.

I was the one being served, royally, by continuing to partake of it. I was also kidding myself, in order to keep doing it. Worse still, I didn't even *know* I was kidding myself!

And while I was busy sneering at non-drinking guy with his soda, I realised with some shame that I did that because his mere presence there caused me to feel uncomfortable, but I mean around my own drinking.

I needed to drink.

He didn't.

I scoffed at him for choosing not to.

He *didn't* jump on his high horse in return. He didn't need to. He was firm and serene in his choices. I wasn't.

I needed validation, and my drinking brain happily obliged.

Except when I was sober.

Well, fuck that. I'll just drink more. Who needs those kinds of thoughts anyway!

3

The Downward Spiral

I'd been drinking for decades by the time I reached this point. My drinking started around the time I first had sex at age 14; it made it possible in fact. And from that early point, my good and willing drinking brain created a strong neural link – alcohol and sex.

The two went together like peas and carrots.

But interestingly, while I found I could drink and not have sex, I certainly could not have sex without drinking.

In fact, I'll go one further, and say that my first sexual experience when my age was still in the single digits – that old story of incest *(the game the whole family can play, some grub once joked with me)* – if I could've drank to blot it out, I would've! But back then, I didn't even know what alcohol did.

Well, that's kind of untrue. I did know.

My dad was a rampant alcoholic, and my earliest memories of him are his red, shiny face, clutching his big smudgy wine goblet, filled to the brim with cheap, stinky red, and directing lewd comments at me when he wasn't hurling abuse. I guess I knew already at that tender age that alcohol *changed* people.

But I didn't understand the mechanics of drinking, or why it was used, and how it also blotted out the drinker's memory afterwards. So, there went any chance of accountability right there - a concept I couldn't grasp, being a kid, but which brought me heaps of disappointment, distress and uncertainty growing up.

My dad drank for his own reasons, but as a kid, all I knew was that when the wine was on the table, the raging monster or the sullen, brooding beast was present also, and to look out! All to be forgotten – by him, not me – the next morning. Gaslighting at its most existential level.

Rethinking this, I can see now that my life was really touched by alcohol from birth.

It was always present. It was there when my mum would get belted up of a night, or when I copped it, or my brother did. It was present when I was sexually interfered with.

As I write this, I can't remember a *single good time* as a kid where the substance was present. It was all bad, bad, bad.

So, those were my beginnings with the social substance.

I started my drinking proper (by societal standards) at around age 18. It was the early 1980s, and booze buses were practically non-existent – so there was no deterrence. Everyone I knew drove drunk, and really thought nothing of it. It was considered a win if you arrived home without a new dent on your car, or you'd not been picked up by a traffic cop for weaving all over the road.

It was also the era of just throwing your rubbish out your car window, and we even made a game of seeing what we could target with our discarded beer cans. My personal favourite was trying to unload a whole bag of McDonalds wrappers out the window with enough precision to land on the windscreen of the car behind us.

It was a different world – a world where all the dangers weren't delineated for you, the way they are now. There was no 'Drink Responsibly,' or little pregnant silhouetted reminders on your stubby of beer, or even 'If you drink and drive, you're a bloody idiot' billboards to remind you what a bloody idiot you were in fact being.

You were free to make your own bad choices – as free as you were to suffer the consequences, depending on how Fate decided to roll its dice that day.

The drinking ebbed and flowed through my life. It was heavy in my early 20s, and then I met my future husband at age 24, and spent the next 13 years mostly *not* drinking. We did partake a little early on, but it always seemed to lead to fights, and if not fights, truly awful hangovers. We drank shit things like UDLs because they tasted like soft drink, and it took nothing to suck down 15 of those in a night. So, apart from the alcohol, you'd ingest roughly half a cubic metre of sugar in those cans.

You never woke up feeling flash afterwards.

The drinking mostly stopped though after the first couple of years of marriage, and in due course we had our daughter, and not too many more moons had passed before we separated and later divorced.

I was then a single mother of a toddler, and being super responsible (as children of alcoholics often are) I didn't partake in drinking around her. In fact, I kind of lost interest in it altogether.

Remember what I said earlier about drinking and sex? Well, there was no sex happening, and therefore there was no need to drink. It's obvious to me now that I never drank for the taste of it. That was just a concept that my drinking brain created for me, so I could binge drink later in life, with the unchallenged belief that I just *loved* the stuff.

As my daughter grew up, and the 'every second weekend with her dad' thing became the norm, those off weekends largely became booze fests with friends. I was kicking up my heels, relishing my short window of irresponsible freedom, and boy did I give it a push! It wasn't too problematic back then though – I just had to ensure I was in good condition by Sunday night, when my daughter returned home from her dad's.

It would be a funny head space I was in, that I never really analysed at the time. But there'd always be this sense of relief when I collected her, knowing that I wouldn't, or couldn't drink like that again for a while. Nobody to impress. I had my daughter to care for, I was a responsible mum, and that was that.

So, Drinking Me would take a time out for the next 12 days, until the next bender.

I just didn't know how to enjoy my time off any other way.

It didn't help that I'd start those free weekends by going to pubs and nightclubs, and drinking copious amounts of piss to even cope with being in those places. That would set the tone for spending the rest of the weekend dealing with the fallout, because as a fortnightly binge drinker, I wasn't 'match-fit.' We used to joke that I needed to get in training, and that I was too much of a lightweight.

Nobody else seemed to have the sort of hangovers I did. But it never occurred to me that perhaps nobody else *admitted* they had them. Because that then would also be truthfully acknowledging they'd drank too much, meaning they'd (heaven forbid) lost control.

The drinkers that admit this kind of behaviour are super rare, as I eventually found out.

Alcohol is not, and never was, a substance of honesty. It's an activity the lower self likes to partake in – and it goes hand in hand with unconsciously lying about it. Or perhaps forgetting about it.

I guess it doesn't matter, really, because the result is the same. It just means you often don't realise you've got a problem - until you can no longer ignore it - and by then, it's generally a big, horribly entrenched problem!

Over the years, my social substance chose my men for me as well – but it tended to choose badly. In fact, it *always* chose badly. I would end up with mentally sick men, jealous men, violent men, addicted men – but never, ever did I end up with an emotionally healthy partner. Most of them I met in drinking environments, and always at least one of us was drunk – usually me – to facilitate the beginning of yet another pointless relationship, doomed to failure.

However, because I'm so unilaterally brilliant at reframing my issues, I came to the conclusion over the years that the *relationships* were the problem. Not my drinking. I would continue to drink. I'd just get rid of him – until I'd find another him. Or rather, he found me.

And so it went on.

When I moved to Queensland with my daughter in my late 40s, my drinking really came into its own. I stepped (leapt) out of my comfort zone, and I took over the running of a singles social club.

Make that a singles drinking club that socialised. Because to my irritation, it quickly became infamous, and sneered at by those outside of the sloshed partying sanctum. You know, those boring folk that apparently could hold their liquor, or didn't drink, and looked down on the fun we were having in our group. *'The group run by a piss-head'* was the general whisper around town, and though I didn't like the label, I went all out to show those judgy assholes that our group of piss-heads had way more fun than anyone else!

And I had plenty of company. At one stage, we had two social groups in our small town, running parallel events; the other group would be attended by the sedate bunch, and then you'd have our events, with roughly four times as many attendees, all being loud and loaded. And I was queen of that group. I made it happen.

Sober Me would plan events, but those events always contained the probability of alcohol. And it didn't matter if the events were in alcoholic environments or not. I could turn a kayaking event into a drinking paddle, or a beach walk into a boozy picnic. It always involved ingesting some alcohol either during, or after the event. And in my case, often prior as well!

You see, my shaky self-confidence needed to load up a little before putting on my 'life of the party' cape, turning on that beaming smile, and hugging and kissing all those people I didn't even know if I liked at all. But nobody ever knew it. All they knew was that good old Caz had arrived on the scene, had created the most amazing social life for them, and if she got a bit messy at times, well, she was a *fun drunk*, so who cared.

I look back now at those times, and realise how little presence I actually felt. Someone would come up, hug me, and I'd invite them in with a big 'How the hell *are* you?' Then I'd watch their lips move in reply – *who the fuck cares how you are* - while I thought up my next witty response. My hand would be firmly curled around my glass too – I noticed I never let it go. It was my lifeline.

All I'd be thinking about was what a great buzz I was having, how I could get all these people along to my events – *Me*, who in my sober state really didn't know how to be a friend to anyone, least of all to myself. And I'd awkwardly brush off compliments from people about how I'd changed their lives, by running this amazing group.

I wasn't selfless like that. I was doing it for me. They just couldn't see it. Maybe because they were drinkers too.

It was bloody exhilarating – and exhausting.

I had nights where I didn't even know how I got home.

I remember one morning clearly, where I woke up to a silent apartment – and my immediate thought was I'd lost my phone. I managed to drag myself off the bed, and hunt around a little for it. Oh, there it is. Good. And my wallet. Double good. And my keys. Yay!

My jacket is gone. Oh well, it's the fourth one I've lost this month – I'll just have to find a place where I can buy denim jackets in bulk, no problem.

I made a coffee, then went back to bed, my brain still marinating uneasily, trying to remember the night.

I knew I'd been to see an AC/DC covers band at the surf club. And I knew I'd met a guy called Mal, who was from Melbourne. And beyond that – no idea. How I got home, how I even managed to leave with my belongings, or who I did or didn't say goodbye to.

I glanced across at the pillow next to me – and wondered if anyone else had been in the bed. I sniffed the sheets. Yes, I did that too. But I had no real answers – until my phone pinged, and there's a message from Mal – I must have given him my contact details – and the dear man filled in some of those blanks for me.

He had walked me home, had got me here safely. *He* was a gentleman. I had apparently asked him to stay – but he had been a gentleman, and said no. And he was now checking to see if I was okay.

Mal is a true gem. And it's why I never saw him again.

Things really began to change when my daughter hit her difficult years around age 14. By then, I'd hooked up with another heavy drinker, Max; a local good-time boy, who'd conveniently hidden the fact he was a bankrupt. And in no time, he'd moved himself, uninvited, into my house. It started with leaving a few work shirts for me to launder, and then suddenly I was doing his work invoices (for free of course) and my daughter was withdrawing more and more.

I began to drink more openly and frequently, now that I had an in-house drinking buddy, and I was mortified because my daughter got to see me really, really drunk, possibly for the first time ever. But I couldn't stop, not when I was having so much fun at last! And I justified it all by telling myself I'd sacrificed my whole life for my daughter, and now she had to fit in her life around me, not vice versa.

(This gem came from one of my wine-loving friends, whose relationship with her own kids was shaky at best). But I took it onboard. Anything to keep drinking.

So, my daughter withdrew more and more (I can see this so clearly now, but couldn't – or wouldn't - then) and decided to move two states away to live with her dad. And Max then asked me to marry him (after 7 weeks!) and I said yes – knowing that this proposal's chance of actually coming to fruition was probably less than zero, but enjoying the spectacle it made within the group.

I didn't even like him that much. But the performance was all that mattered.

So, when I hit my big 5-0, I finally felt I had it all. I had the massive party I'd waited my whole life for. I was living the dream in Noosa, Queensland. I had a good-looking bloke, that most of the town had already slept with and discarded – and which I refused to believe. And most importantly, I had my beer. To make all the other things work – most notably and painfully, the absence of my daughter.

I have a photo book of that 50th birthday party onboard the Noosa Queen, a lovely old river boat. There's a band, including my non-drinking brother who'd flown up for the occasion. There's me singing (screeching) into a microphone. I don't remember doing that, but it was part of the fantasy depicted in the memento photo album. I'm surprised people weren't wearing earmuffs in those happy snaps.

And then there's not *one* cake – but *two*! One is my birthday cake. And the other just has a Nike tick on it and says 'JUST DO IT' – and that was my engagement cake – for Mr and Mrs Spontaneously Sloshed. My best friend Denise had organised these things for me – God bless one of the only non-drinking friends I ever had that genuinely liked me, either drunk or sober. And still does.

So, there's the two flashy cakes – and the photos are all of me clutching stubbies of beer, with my drunk fiancé. This was our Magic Moment. And after that moment, we made more moments by moving the party to my cute little house, which pretty much got trashed from holding fifty-odd drunks and a band, when it was designed to house maybe a family of four and a dog.

Now, I'd like to say we all rode happily off into the sunset after that day – but you already know that it didn't turn out like that, don't you? Life doesn't flow for you when you have that much alcohol in your life - it *never* ends up like that.

The relationship faltered, like so many others. And I went back to running the group, presenting that smiling front – except I wasn't smiling so much anymore.

Well, I'd *start* the nights off that way, preloaded on drink, but it more and more frequently ended in tears – mine – as the alcohol started to insidiously bring up childhood traumas for me. And these tears would spill out at the most inconvenient times.

I even had a good friend state to my partner at the time, 'Why do you bother with her, she's just feeling sorry for herself. She's hard work; and you deserve so much better,' which really infuriated me. Because I couldn't even argue - it was a legitimate assessment of me.

I was in full-blown victim mode by then, and Drinking Brain was simply running amok during those binges. The shame afterwards was almost unbearable.

And it really was becoming very messy indeed. I was drinking more and more, and worse still, starting to mix drinks, like shots and beer and wine, in fact, pretty much anything that was going. People in our group would supply home brew, the real cheap and nasty stuff, in order for us drunks to save money. And having no off button, this culminated in some benders that

I often feared I would not recover from.

Worse still, I wondered why I didn't even seem to care anymore, bar how physically awful I felt.

Something – something – had to give.

4

The Final Drinking Years

A reprieve finally came from an unexpected quarter. Having drank, sobbed, partied and regretted my way through the remainder of 2016, an opportunity came through my daughter, who lived with her dad in another state at the time. I had found myself increasing my visits with her, as her relationship with her dad and his partner deteriorated. I didn't know how much of it was the same teen angst I'd experienced before she left me two years prior – but by believing that, I gave myself the green light to carry on drinking in the interim. I'd tried to coax her back to Queensland, but her father wouldn't allow her to, taunting me with 'You can't just change your mind now – she's got *stability* here with us.'

Yeah. Right.

Seeing my daughter in pain, seemingly trapped in that situation, and after she'd already been forced to make starts at three different high schools, I was loath to step in in any real sense of the word. Plus my ex had sneered at me to, 'Just keep drinking, Caz,' and that was one suggestion of his that I had no trouble cooperating with!

I was on a visit to Melbourne in November 2016 when the shit really hit the fan - but this time I was there, and present for a change. I had ceased drinking for what I hoped was the last time – it turned out it wasn't – but by the time I was there that November, I had about three months of sobriety behind me. I know now though that what I was was a 'dry drunk' – that curious state where a drinker still wants to drink, but has managed to stay off the substance on a willpower basis. Willpower being what it is, dry drunks always eventually get soaked again when the conditions present themselves.

So there was I, witnessing the 'stable family situation' unravel spectacularly right before my eyes in Melbourne, and my daughter in floods of hysterical tears, wearing her one tatty school dress. And as I held her and tried to soothe her, I faced a monumental dilemma that was going on in my head.

Mother Heart was saying, 'This can't go on. I need to return to Melbourne for my daughter's final year of school. It's so important; her whole future depends on it. There's no stability here at all! *I can see it now with my own eyes.*' But drinking brain was whispering, *'You won't be able to drink, though. Think of the summer in Noosa, with all your friends. I know you're not drinking at the moment - but it's not forever. You're just having a break. Imagine being stuck down in Melbourne for a year, with no partying - and don't forget those long, depressing winters. And you'll be living in the northern suburbs too, so no friends to party with! There's not even a beach to keep you sane. Just keep quiet, and things will settle down. You're out of here in a few days. Just go home, and go back to your life in Queensland. She'll cope. After all, YOU coped with far worse as a kid.'*

I continued to hold her little sobbing body, while I privately mulled over what a year spent undrinking would entail, while doing what was morally the right thing. I could rent a unit near the school for the year. Most importantly, I could be the mother I wished I had have been two years ago, when I'd lost my way because of the drinking and partying. I couldn't change what had gone on back then, but I could redeem myself now.

It was my opportunity to right the wrongs, I realised – if I had the courage.

Before I knew it, my lips were murmuring, 'Don't worry, sweetheart. I'm going to move back to Melbourne for the next year, and you're going to live with me while you finish high school.' The words came out even before I'd had a chance to digest them. But I didn't regret them. Especially when I felt her stiffen momentarily in my arms, and then the next few words that came out, the most heartfelt words I'd heard in a long time – simply, 'Oh Mummy.... *Really*?' The voice was so quiet, so tearfully hopeful – and yet so scared I didn't mean it. And I responded then with a firm, 'Absolutely! This can't go on. I'm going to find us a place. But please don't change your mind, because I'll have to sign a lease for a year.'

I didn't know this at the time, but my daughter told me afterwards that her brain was doing elated back flips, to the tune of - *You've got to be kidding* – AS IF *I'd change my mind! This is amazing!*

So, I finally got a break. Or more importantly, my three months sobriety gave me enough perspective and courage to take the break when it came.

#

I wish I could say 2017 was spent in a gloriously sober state – but alas, this is no fairy tale. I was eight months sober at the time I fell off the wagon in around May 2017, and it was by no means a conscious decision to start drinking again. But alcohol is like that – it awaits its opportunity, and here it was.

I was attending a music event at a local club called Musicland. The name sounds like a theme park, ostensibly for all things musical – but of course music goes with drinking. Doesn't everything?

Musicland became my local hang-out, my weekend party venue. The first time I went, I drank coke and water, and felt a bit socially awkward. The second time, I decided I could have just one beer. After all, I had been sober for so long now, I was sure I was firmly in control.

I gazed at the drinks fridge. Sober brain alarmedly said I should perhaps choose a light beer; that's of course if I really *had* to drink. But drinking brain licked its lips and slyly suggested I go for my old favourite, Carlton Draught. Full strength, heavy, lush. And because they were the same price, and because clearly I was just a dry drunk at that stage, drinking brain won. Not that there was much of a battle.

I drank that Carlton Draught – and it tasted like kaka. But by the time I got halfway through it, I had a bit of a buzz happening, and so I forced myself to finish it, still disliking the taste. And then no more. I felt triumphant, and in control. *I could have just one!*

Drinking brain remained smugly silent. It needed no further commentary – because it had managed to get its foot back in the door. As for me, I then drank copious amounts of water, noting it took a surprising amount of time to completely sober up. And then I drove home – because those days I could drive everywhere. For a little while longer, anyway.

The next week I was back there again - and had another

Carlton Draught. Except this time, I'd brought my personal breathalyser with me – just so I could check. Drinking brain had quietly popped it into the car for me. After all, it wouldn't do to get caught drink driving now, would it? So, having had that one beer, I did a reading, then looked at the time - and figured I could easily have a second beer, eat some food – and *still* be okay to drive home.

So, I did.

The breathalyser informed me that I still had some alcohol in my system when I started driving, but I was below the legal limit – and besides I couldn't wait all night for it to drop down to a nil reading. The nights were getting cold, and the temperature would get to zero before I could!

And so it went on. Until just a few weeks later, I remember sitting in my daughter's little Mazda (I usually drove her car to Musicland) repeatedly and impatiently breathalysing, and wishing I hadn't drank *quite* so much. My blood alcohol reading was taking forever to drop to the legal driving limit.

So I sat there, huddled in a blanket that drinking brain had now thoughtfully provided be kept in the car (so I could stay warm whilst sobering up of course) – and wondered how on earth I was back, doing this shit again. I felt like crying.

This went on for a while. I'd have a whale of a time, not drinking to my capacity though, otherwise I'd be spending whole nights in the car. But what I did start doing was taking my campervan to Musicland instead, so I had a bit of comfort to sober up in.

I remember one night, meeting another soul who had his campervan there too – and I recall how we both laughed about being kings of the universe for having that kind of forethought. It reminded me of my mate Sam in Queensland, who I'd had similar conversations with. He too drove a mobile bed, and for the same reason. It wasn't to camp - it was an essential conveyance no serious drinker would ever want to be without! And along with the bed, it contained things like water, headache pills, snacks – and even a toilet. The drinker's recovery kit. Which made the whole process so much more comfortable.

But things of course got messy. There was some weird fellow I used to dance with there, who was always harassing me for more, and was quite touchy feely when we did dance. There was a sound technician who I think I'd had a drunken pash with one night, who couldn't seem to forget it, and I'd spy him up there in the sound booth, giving me gooey, wistful looks which made me shudder. And then there was the night I copped a drink spike.

I didn't realise it at the time. But I'd arrived there, had a couple of drinks, and ran into this weasel I knew from a social group I'd joined at the venue. And suddenly, mystifyingly, I was legless, smashed off my tits drunk. It was so early in the night that half the regulars I knew there had only just arrived. I greeted one of them with a tongue down the throat (I only have a very sketchy memory of this, mostly because he good-naturedly told me about it afterwards, and I trust him) and then the next thing that happened was I was out the front of the venue, throwing my guts up, and the weasel was conveniently offering to drive me home. What a sterling fellow he turned out to be. I'm told he's currently serving time in jail for date rape and assault.

But I digress.

I don't remember much of that trip. What I do remember is him having to pull up a few times so I could repeatedly throw up. And I *never* throw up. I have a vague memory of him making sexual innuendos towards me, but me being too sick and drunk to care. And having arrived at home, I recall staggering upstairs and crashing into bed. Where I remained for two days. I felt incredibly ill, and I realised that this was no regular hangover.

Over the ensuing period, I had friends contacting me, concerned about how drunk I'd been. Join the club! I couldn't work out why I'd been so drunk either – but then a friend suggested to me that my drink may have been spiked.

As a drinker, I'd always dismissed the idea of drink spiking – even though I was such a target for it. I'd leave my open drinks anywhere and everywhere, whenever I'd suddenly leap up to dance. So this was really an incident waiting to happen, and the biggest surprise was it took as long as it did.

I was also horrified when that slimy weasel contacted me on Messenger the next day, ostensibly to see how I was, but then went on to tell me what a marvellous looking rack I had, and how sexy I was, on the way home.

It was enough to make me hurl all over again.

Alas are the perils of drinking. And I was there, back at square one, hating myself, miserable as all fuck – and wondering how it had all ended up like this again. I couldn't even talk to anyone about it, so ashamed was I to have put myself in such a position.

But you don't think of the possible repercussions when you're drinking like that. Drinking brain does not look out for you. Drinking brain just wants to drink.

#

I finished my stint in Melbourne at the end of 2017 – and my daughter moved back in with her dad, because I was returning to Queensland. I felt I'd done the right thing for that year, but in truth I was pretty messed up.

I was a binge drinker again – and was looking forward to going back north, to drink 'safely' with my old friends. I clearly had a short memory, as it was with those same friends that I'd had the mother of all benders back in 2016, where I'd drank that much I thought I was going to die. That was the bender that had resulted in the eight months of sobriety afterwards.

But drinking brain doesn't hang onto those kinds of lessons. Drinking brain keeps egging you on in the hope you do in fact die one day.

I was one of the lucky ones – I'm still here.

However, drinking brain hadn't finished with me yet.

I returned to Queensland, got started on renovating a house I'd bought sight unseen whilst in Melbourne – and partying. Until suddenly early in 2018, a mere six weeks after arriving home, I got a terrified phone call from my daughter, telling me her dad had suddenly died. At age 55. Heart attack. And as it turned out, he'd become a heavy drinker of red in his last years – but I only learned this after the fact.

I did, however, have a few indignant moments, recalling how he'd shamed *me* about *my* drinking! But I guess he got to have the last word about that, if nothing else.

Rest in peace, Mick.

The next two years were a non-stop backwards and forwards between Melbourne and Queensland, supporting my daughter, and then alternating it with indulging in the Queensland partying lifestyle.

It was like I was split in two, living a double life. And interspersed in all this, I inadvertently met a partner, Michael, at a camping (drinking) event I was running.

The next while went by in a blur, with him and without him – flying to Melbourne, time in Queensland, lots of cruises (Michael loved these the same way I did) and just overall increased alcoholic messiness as time went on. Twice as messy, given we were *both* big drinkers.

I began having some serious meltdowns too, in between the bouts of drinking.

I had spread myself so thin, you see.

Not only was I committed to financing my daughter's household until some money from her dad's estate came in, I was actively engaged in a lawsuit, whilst somehow holding down a job myself, paying my own two mortgages, and partnering another heavy drinker with his own unique set of behavioural issues.

We'd also bought a unit together – and then a house – and then ran an Airbnb – all the while partnering, breaking up, and repartnering.

We even had a dog at some stage that Michael had acquired from his auntie in South Australia when he was there one time, feeling suicidal, and which some months later needed to be returned as an inconvenience when it was no longer required once we repartnered.

So – something had to give. Again.

I won't bore you with too much detail – I probably already have!

For me, the final crunch came at last on 13 December 2019, after we'd had our final 'fun' drinking session. I'd sobbed my heart out yet again, Michael was bewildered, and I pushed him away once more. I knew I'd mortally wounded not only his heart, but my own.

I dropped him off at a bus stop in Melbourne, around the corner from my pad in St Kilda. And as I drove away, I glanced across the road to where he stood, looking forlornly down at his phone. I saw the hurt and the pain, etched in his body language. And I finally realised I could not go on.

I was at the end of the road. I could not hurt this person anymore. Or myself.

Especially myself.

I had had my last drink.

Over the next few days, quietly reflecting, alone, the decision finally solidified for me that alcohol must have no part in my life going forward. And if that meant the relationship was a casualty of my not drinking – so be it.

Nothing was worth the price we were both paying to keep drinking.

I realised the sole responsibility of this decision rested heavily on myself – but I was also my solution. And I was finally going to change my life.

So, that's my back story – the why.

Now let's move on, to the what, and the how. And the now.

5

The Fucking Lie That Is Alcohol

Let's start this by having a look at alcohol from a different angle, beginning with the Fucking Lie That Is Alcohol.

Let's shine the light of Truth on the beast.

It's the big, pissed elephant in the room of your world view.

It sits there, watching you struggle in its grip, like a fly caught in a deadly sticky web.

But it wasn't always this way, was it?

Well, unfortunately, it was – for some of us.

Let's visit a couple of households, where that elephant runs amok, always in the background - till it's front and centre stage.

Let's see how those kids get to grow up.

Maybe your childhood was a bit like this – or maybe it was different.

But just for educational purposes, let's call in at that ordinary looking house in the next street.

#

The child is playing on her backyard swing. She's a pretty little creature, hair hanging in blond ringlets in a kind of uncared-for permanent wave, like long tassled ropes either side of her thin, grubby face. Her eyes are light blue; alert, questioning. They focus on every sight and every sound.

To an adult, that back yard is a wasteland of dry red dirt, peppered with big thistles. To the child though, and her younger brother, it's an adventure wonderland they explore every day.

From inside the house come raucous voices, and the regular sounds of clinking glasses. Some laughter. Sometimes it sounds more like screaming.

It's getting a bit cold now – the wind has picked up, and the sky is darkening already, even though it's only four o'clock.

The child decides to look for her brother.

'*Alfie,*' she calls in her thin little bleat – but the wind hijacks it off behind the thistles. She climbs off the swing, and after ascertaining her little brother is nowhere in sight, she bounds blithely up the back steps into the house. She almost trips over her mother, who is wiping something off the linoleum by the back door.

There is a reeky, unpleasant smell.

'Oh, look out, stupid child!' complains her mother, discombobulated by the girl's sudden clumsy appearance. And then, 'Oh, wait!' – and the gnarled hand reaches out to snatch the tottering wine glass that the child's foot has just brushed in passing. But not quickly enough – the glass falls over.

It's a dead soldier, spilling its lifeblood over the already sticky floor.

THE FUCKING LIE THAT IS ALCOHOL

The child feels a resounding *whop!* in the back of the head, such that her ears feel like they're exploding, under attack. The next angry words leave her in no doubt.

'You clumsy little asshole! Why don't you ever look where you're going! *Now* look what you've done!'

The child, sobbing, holding her hands over her shocked cranium, peering through her hands at her mother – whose eyes are now boring into hers, red and wet and angry.

Mummy's been crying. Again.

'But Mummy – I can't find – ' - - -

Another whack, this one surprising the child from behind.

It's her father – and *he* is someone she *never* wants to get in the way of.

'Stupid little cunt,' he mutters, as he wrenches the fridge open to pull another beer. He glances at the mayhem in the kitchen. '*Two* stupid cunts,' he amends – burps – and then shambles back to the lounge, dragging the remains of a six-pack.

The smaller cunt looks at the big, teary cunt wiping the mess off the floor – and realises with relief that all is as usual. It's just another day.

The child goes back down the stairs into the yard, to look for Alfie.

#

(In another town – another time – another place:)

'*No! No! Mummy!!!*' shrieks the small boy, in a kind of hysteria. Tears pour from his huge, dark eyes as he implores his mother, who's sitting on the couch, red-faced, a glass in front of her. *I don't like Daddy touching me!* Her eyes look at him, glazed, indifferent.

He doesn't want me to –' begins Dad, looking over at Mum.

She snaps, 'It's *your* fucking turn! I change him all day long.'

She takes another big slug, indifferent to the child's irritatingly loud screams.

Dad picks up his yelling son, and roughly slaps the boy down onto the change table, throwing over his shoulder *'You were the one wanted all these fuckin' kids.'*

He pulls at the little tabs securing the nappy around the tiny, thrashing legs. It pulls away, and the child screams as if being murdered.

Dad gives him a shake, enough to make his little jaws rattle.

'Calm down, you little fucker. You think I'm doing this for fun?? Calm the fuck down, I tell you!'

The child lies still, momentarily forgetting to cry.

Dad takes a long, gulping swig from his bottle – and the child suddenly says 'Bot-bot?'

The father swallows, and sneers. 'You want some? Okay – cop this!' and he pours a quantity into the child's open mouth. The child gurgles and resumes his sobbing.

Dad laughs.

You're just a waste of good beer.

He glances at his screaming son with distaste, then uses a wipe to carelessly swipe the child's bottom. The child only howls harder.

Dad burps, and then refastens the same nappy onto the child and heads back to the kitchen, pausing to drop the screaming child into his playpen on the way.

#

(And in another household, this one far, far away, up in the opulent Hills District:)

It was Madeline's birthday party, and she was six. It was very exciting. She'd only started primary school that year, so this was her first 'big kid' party. She'd invited six girls from school, promising them there'd be a pink cake, and fairy costumes, and games.

Madeline's friends gazed with amazement at the huge house, pretty with streamers and balloons in pastel shades.

They were almost too excited to eat the fairy bread. And as for the *champagne* – there were the palest pink lemonades, six to a tray, all lined up in fancy glass flutes.

Madeline's mother, clutching her own lipstick-stained flute, was passing the tray amongst the little girls.

'Time to celebrate,' she cooed.

The girls exclaimed in wonderment and giggles, as they took their glasses.

'Now – wait everybody! – now – wait - CHEERS!' shrieked Mother, and she clashed her glass against that of Madeline.

Dad fired off the happy snaps on his phone, trying to juggle the task with his own can of Tooheys, and clapping at the same time. It was no mean feat – but he captured a substandard memory.

The girls all giggled, and mightily encouraged, began clinking and clashing their own glasses with each other, over and over and over and over.

High on sugar, and pink champagne in fancy flutes, the kids agreed with Mother that they'd had the best time ever. And best of all, Mother was telling Madeline she was the most beautiful birthday girl today, and *so grown up now*!

Madeline beamed. It had been the best day ever for her too.

#

Nobody was *born* with a glass of alcohol in their hand. But we were all born into a society that values drinking. Some would argue it's a society that *needs* drinking, in order to escape life, with all its ups and downs, at least momentarily. Until that escape can sometimes become, unnoticed, a regular event.

I guess that perspective depends on what kind of life you lead, and how honest you are about it.

We can take it all the way back to before we're born, if you like. Yeah, let's start there. Come with me – the labour ward is this way.

Here's Mum-to-be – and for the sake of seeing the full context here, let's start at the pregnancy. You get told, especially in the first trimester, that you shouldn't drink alcohol, as that's when the framework for the emerging new life is under construction, as well as its growth environment. Which is fine – but unless you *know* the moment you're pregnant, you *don't know* to stop drinking right at that point.

If Mum-to-be is a regular drinker, she will have imbibed a considerable amount before even discovering there's this new life growing inside of her.

Nevertheless, in a less-than-ideal world, she then abstains from drinking alcohol, at least until that child is born into the world. Ditto with smoking, that other addiction I'm not covering in this book.

But you get the idea. Most women want to give their baby a fighting chance.

Of course, the general consensus was – but hopefully still isn't - that it's really *only* that first trimester we should abstain from alcohol, and then after that, well, it's still not a *good* thing, but a glass here or there probably won't matter too much.

Now, I don't know what the majority of pregnant women decide on that basis, whether to drink or not to drink – but it's a fair argument that the foetus has probably been exposed to at least *some* alcohol over that nine months.

Moving on to post-natal drinking behaviour - it's my experience that women who were problem drinkers prior to giving birth, don't find life suddenly less stressful as a new parent, such that they no longer need to drink.

Quite the opposite in fact – huge life changes can be incredibly stressful.

And early wiring, for that new child, is dynamite. Medical science agrees that much of the child's behavioural wiring is formed in the first seven years of life.

So, let's now brainstorm some of the things that that child might ingest during those early formative years.

Perhaps Mum and Dad are under the pump financially – often new parents are.

Perhaps they use a drink or drinks at night to unwind.

They might then have friends over on the weekend to watch the footy, and cheer and drink. The kids might watch the footy with them. And they see the ads for alcohol on the big screen. They might even notice it's the same brand that Daddy drinks. And adults always seem to be so *happy* with that drink in their hand, don't they?

Look at Mum and Dad there, with all their friends – and they're *all drinking beer*.

Having a blast!

The kids might fetch Dad another beer, when asked.

Meanwhile, Mum and her friends, all clutching elegant-looking wine glasses, are giggling in the kitchen about something. They look happy too!

Sometimes Mum and Dad even get all lovey-dovey with each other – which is sort of icky, but a lot better than some of the fights the kids overhear later on.

Those seem to happen, now and then, after those happy, long drinking afternoons, when the footy is over and the friends have gone home.

But it had seemed like such a good day. It's very confusing – and unpredictable.

By the time a child gets to primary school, there will have been a presence of alcohol around them in some way, either directly in the home, or when out and about. And of course, they'll have seen the ads on TV, and the constant presence of alcohol in the movies they watch. And these days, of course, it's all over social media as well.

All designed, of course, to normalise the demon drink in our lives from the earliest age. Glamourise it, even, as a desirable part of adult life.

And most kids don't wait to become an adult before they're trying it on for size themselves – with no idea of what they're playing with.

But let the party start!

Some people even regard alcohol as a collectable. They'll have wine cellars, or if they haven't got one of those, they'll display racks and racks of it, sometimes in their living rooms. Like being a wine snob is some kind of badge of honour.

Or there will be a bar in the house that will contain all manner of spirits and liquors, just for when guests come over, they say. Or Dad will have a fridge full of beer out in the back garage – and the reason it's out there is because he has so damn much of it that it would swamp the indoor fridge and leave no room for things like food.

Alcohol takes up a lot of space, especially when it's bought in bulk.

And why is it bought in such quantities? Because it's *cheaper* that way!

It doesn't matter if the chosen poison is beer or wine, it's the same. It's cheaper to buy a dozen bottles of wine than buy it by the one or two. It's cheaper to buy two slabs of beer, than buy it by the six pack. And what does that matter – because it makes good sense, doesn't it? After all, it's not like it's going to go to waste.

Alcohol is a regular *staple*, and if the only way you can get it cheap is by buying it in bulk – well, it's the same for food, right?

That's why we have Costco and the like. Or Dan Murphy's, Liquorland, or Celebrations.

Heavy drinkers are economists – and that's because they need to be. Daily drinking can be darn expensive!

(Note: since when was alcohol regarded as a "staple"?)

As a side note – let's look at some of the names of these places.

Liquor Legends (is that what drinking makes me?)

Cellarbrations (yippee, I'm pissing away my money on alcohol again!)

First Choice Liquor Mart.

Super Cellars.

Liquorland (sounds like a bloody theme park).

Star Liquor (*you're* a star for choosing *us*).

Thirsty Camel (I'm parched – you must be too!)

Bob's Bulk Booze.

And good old Dan Murphy's (affectionately referred to as the Uncle Dan's of our warm, fuzzy, drinking family.)

It makes me wonder – why aren't they called things like -

Hangover Heaven?

Fatty Liverland, anyone?

How about Cirrhosis Cellars -

or even DV Drinks?

Truth in advertising just doesn't sell the dream the same way though, does it?

What are your early childhood memories around alcohol?

Let me share mine with you.

I remember as a kid being confused a lot of the time, around the uncertainty of Dad's mood swings. One minute he'd be fine, cooing all over me – and the next he'd be swearing at us, or belting my mother, or coming after my brother and I.

But of course, at that age, how could I put two and two together?

I know I grew to hate the smell of red wine. I still do, after all this time. It smells like pure evil to me.

As a kid, I somehow knew the stuff was bad, even if I didn't know it was the reason for the mood swings. It just always seemed to be present when things turned ugly.

I grew up to ads everywhere for beer and for smoking. I thought the Marlborough Man was cool. I remember the ads for Fosters Lager, and Vic Bitter. And the movies I watched all seemed to show adults drinking in them, and looking all the more happy and glamorous for doing so.

Drinking somehow made bored housewives into the bold and the beautiful. It made boys into men. It made wrongs right.

And so were the days of their lives.

Dad would have a friend over occasionally – he didn't have many – but those friends were always heavy drinkers and smokers. And in those days, nobody thought anything of doing both in the house, or while driving, for that matter!

We would get driven home from Dad's friend's house, with Dad driving drunk, and Mum shrieking at him. We two kids would be huddled down in the back seat, sans seat belts, as they didn't exist in those days. And although we knew that something bad was happening, and even noticed that Dad's driving seemed to be all over the road - we really had no concept of the danger that was causing Mum to scream the way she did.

Somehow - we survived those trips.

I have memories of Dad entering my bedroom at times, stinking of that evil red wine, and he'd stand at my bedroom door, swaying, and glaring at me.

I never knew why.

I'd be just lying on my bed, quietly reading a book.

Or sometimes, I'd quickly shut my eyes tightly and pretend I was asleep.

I couldn't imagine in what universe that what I was doing was somehow wrong – but it always seemed to be. The only question in my mind would be was it wrong enough to get me punished, and how severely.

I never knew where anyone else in the house was in those moments. Time stood still.

I now know, of course, that it was the demons in his own head, fanned by the red wine coursing through his veins, that caused him to act the way he did. Because he never did this sober.

He was a delightful, and reasonable man when he didn't drink. But sadly, those times were few and far between.

But all misdemeanors were forgotten the next day – his real ones, and my perceived ones.

Everyone would get up and go off to work, we kids would go off to school (my only real sane space as a kid) and then we'd return home in the afternoon, never quite knowing what we were walking into.

Those were the days of *our* lives!

If you're lucky enough to have not grown up in a home touched by alcohol, you, dear reader, are one of the fortunate ones.

But it doesn't give you a free ticket either – and I suspect that's why you're here, reading this book. Because alcohol can touch anyone, even decades down the track.

It did with me.

The problem with normalising alcohol use in front of our children, is we are setting down the foundational building blocks for them – and it's a layer of neural wiring that will be in place for them, ready to build on, as they reach maturity.

Because our kids look up to us, plain and simple.

Even in the midst of our own worst behaviours, they still do that. We are their guiding lights, and their heroes - yes, even when we're unaware they are watching us – and learning, all the time. Taking it in.

Unconscious foundational wiring is such a funny, silent thing. I'm a great example of this. I remember very clearly as I grew up, deciding I would never touch alcohol, the exact mantra in my head being *'I will never be like Dad.'*

Because even at a tender age, I could see Dad hurt people when he drank. He was abusive. He was violent. He drove dangerously. His face fell into unpleasant lines.

The drink was always the common denominator. And even though I had no understanding of how alcohol bent his brain out of shape, just being a kid at that stage, I knew that somehow the substance caused people to do stuff they wouldn't ordinarily do if they weren't drinking.

So, I was never going to do that!

Plus I hated the smell of it, and something that smelt that bad could only taste putrid as well.

Easy decision for me. I'd stick to milkshakes.

Note to self:

If it looks like shit, smells like shit, and tastes like shit – it probably is shit.

Good thing to stay away from it.

Roll forward a decade or so, and sadly but predictably, I'd begun to use alcohol myself.

I remember absolutely hating the taste of it at first. I'd started with Southern Comfort – I remember liking the name of it, maybe it was the comfort aspect – and then some bright spark suggested I mix it with Coke to make it more palatable.

So I did. But all it did was make my Coke taste like shit too.

I then tried beer. That was easier to get down, especially after the first one or two.

But why did I drink?

Well, there were boys, you see.

I never purchased the alcohol myself. I never even went into a bottle shop until decades later. It was always purchased *for* me – and I drank it – so it would facilitate whatever those boys wanted from me.

Again, pretty simple.

They don't call it Leg-Opener for nothing.

Gets back to what I said earlier. You'd never do half the things you do, without the alcohol. But it never sees you doing *good* things.

It is *always* bad things.

Soul destroying stuff.

I don't want to make this book all about me – but I have to draw on myself fearlessly as my own reference point, to share these experiences with you. And what I came to understand, after decades of drinking, is the stuff literally affects every single aspect of your life. All under the guise of 'having fun.'

What I was really having were bad experiences in a vacuum.

Each time, I was numbed to what was occurring, until afterwards – when I literally couldn't look at myself in the mirror.

I grew to hate myself, and what I was doing. And so I drank more – because I no longer knew *how* to be any different.

I was scared there was nothing else *to* me – and maybe there never had been.

Perhaps the drink was all I had, or was.

I was afraid of finding this out for sure.

So, fear kept me drinking. And I beat myself up remorselessly for it – but only when I was sober, of course.

I know it all sounds hopeless. But it isn't – and I'm proof of that.

Here I am, writing this book, at around three and a half years of mostly effortless sobriety.

Life is so damn good now, that I'm writing this book for humanity.

I'm calling out the fucking lie that is alcohol.

I want to scream it from the rooftops, for every kid, every mother, every father, every single person who's suffered under its influence, either directly or indirectly.

And I know my efforts here aren't going to be in vain – because I know that people will read this book – and it's going to help someone. Maybe you.

I'm here to tell you that you're not alone in feeling that alcohol is a big problem. It is. And this little book will be out there in the Universe, long after I'm gone, and may help other souls, sometime in the future.

That's the universal, energetic payoff for me. I've done something worthwhile with my experience.

So with that in mind, I'm going to dive deep now – so take a big breath, and watch me *really* push some buttons.

6

Drinking and Dating

It took me a long, long time to realise that drinking and dating don't go together, at least not in any positive way.

The problem I had was I simply could not imagine going on a dry date, especially with a stranger. And yet that's precisely when you really would want your wits about you, wouldn't you think?

All of my relationships began with drinking – yes, even the current one, which has survived my transition from drunk to dry, but not without its challenges. Still, those challenges were nothing like how hopeless the odds were, had we kept drinking.

But I'm getting ahead.

Meet me at the nightclub in about an hour, okay?

I've got some interesting characters I'd like you to meet.

#

It's 8 pm at our local club, and the big goons who police the door are checking us in, *and checking us out,* as we enter. They're leering at the good-looking sorts, who stagger in on enormous heels – but generally they're just waving us girls through.

They can't tell I've already had a few when I arrive there – I *need* to have a few to even force myself to enter these places. But they don't hassle me yet. They will later.

At this early stage, the goon merely offers me a drinks card as a welcome, which gives me two freebies. I accept it graciously, and will go back to him later on, just a little more flirtatiously, to see if I can score another card off him. And I have a good strike rate.

I see my friend Bob, and I wave, and he saunters over, and casually throws an arm around me in greeting. He tells me I'm getting fat. I tell him to look in the mirror. He then suggests to me I should stop drinking so fast.

I ask him why.

He then shares with me a little story, about how blokes like him operate.

You know, the kind who go to bars to pick up.

He tells me to listen up, so I don't end up a victim that night.

His method, he says, is that he has a drink in front of him, but he sips it very, very slowly. You want to give the *illusion* that you're drinking, he says, but you don't want it affecting you. Bob knows that nobody there will be paying attention to how much he is drinking, or even if he is really drinking at all. But he likes to have an authentic prop, he says.

He isn't there to drink though. He's there to score. And so what he does, he tells me, is he singles out one or two targets that he finds fuckable. Fuckable always means girls who are *drinking without restraint*, and who are becoming *friendlier* as the night wears on.

Looks aren't all that important, even though Bob likes slim

girls – but an easy lay is an easy lay. His target might be dancing in a group of girls, or if she's had a bit more alcohol than the others, she might even be dancing solo, and being a bit outrageous.

Those are Bob's targets. Narrowing them down is easy, he says.

The real art is in knowing when to strike.

When Bob deems that his target has downed enough drink, he will generally approach, and make eye contact. Bob's a good-looking guy, with a nice smile, and he's also a slick dancer. It's quite easy, really. He'll make eye contact, and quite often his target will invite him in with a smile to have a boogie with her -because most blokes don't dance.

(A friend once told me he finally learnt to dance properly because it's a skill that's effectively vertical foreplay, and if you don't do it, your pickings are much slimmer. Yes, I have some interesting friends.)

Once Bob's in there, dancing with his prey, he'll move in a bit closer – but not so close so as to appear sleazy - and then suggest that as they're so hot and sweaty now, would she like a drink?

Free drinks to drunks are like formula to a baby – and of course the idea is met with enthusiasm. Bob escorts her to the bar to choose her poison. He doesn't mind paying for it, he assures her, because thus far he's effectively spent nothing. He was given his own drinks card upon entry, and he uses it now.

It's a darn sight cheaper than paying for sex, he smirks.

Bob's main game was to get the girl to don her beer goggles long enough to want to go home with him - or invite him to her home (better) – and, most importantly, to follow through.

Now, it's not foolproof of course, Bob warns. A better predator might come along and derail his plan. Or if she's drank too much, she might get tired, or emotional, or something other than sexed up.

Balancing the alcohol intake is crucial, he says. But he has a reasonable strike rate.

The main thing is that *without alcohol, he'd have no strike rate at all*.

Another friend, Nick, calls it the wounded gazelle scenario. He told me that when he attends the local nightclub, he'll look for the wounded gazelle. It's the one, he says, that generally isn't as pretty as its herd-mates, and therefore will often be drinking more to compensate.

Then Nick would appear alongside *her* – after watching awhile, in the same hunting style as Bob – and sweep her off her feet with his big smile and good looks.

Nick was also tall, and yes, Nick danced of course. But it was his open wallet at the bar that was the clincher.

The gazelle couldn't believe its luck – and neither could its friends. And having nabbed his prey, Nick would drag her off to the bar to top her up, then waste no time in removing her from the herd so he could finish the job.

Usually in his car, parked conveniently around the back of the club.

I've heard more of these types of tales, but these are by no means exceptional blokes. They just operate in a similar fashion.

One that works.

So, every Friday or Saturday night, lots and lots of girls end up having sex with lots and lots of men that alcohol has basically chosen for them. Because a sober girl wouldn't do it.

In fact, if a sober girl is in a place like this, it's often only because she's the designated driver. And you bet she won't be going home with anybody!

Nor will she even be approached by these kinds of blokes.

One on one dating is a little different, of course - but the drinking is no less crucial.

Two sober people, meeting for the first time on a date, are likely to be respectful, and perhaps a little awkward. Neither of those qualities will lead to spontaneous, unconsidered sex, which may then spawn an ill-conceived relationship.

So that's why the alcohol is important there too. It's why most dates occur over drinks, or dinner and drinks.

It gets the party started before anyone can realise that they don't even actually want to party with that other person.

If you've ever watched "reality" shows like Married At First Sight, or The Bachelor, or First Dates, you'll notice there's an *ocean* of alcohol involved. But it's never, ever mentioned, not by the experts - goodness no! Or indeed even by anyone that's actually *doing* the drinking on those shows, and nor by those people being paid to film the mayhem.

It's just universally accepted that drinking alcohol is a requirement, to fuel the flirt factor, but also the truly atrocious behaviour that will be captured for the nation's viewing pleasure.

Try to imagine how those reality shows would go in a dry environment – it would be comical, because nothing would even get started. And also, it's just not reality, is it, for people to date without drinking.

But getting on to relationships – this is where I'll get to my own experience – and I have a little. I've never struggled getting *into* relationships, but what I've struggled with is *getting out* of them.

Because as a drinker, I was always fair game.

Even later in life, as I became way more discerning – but probably menopausal – and became far less interested in engaging in the horizontal mambo, I still attracted drinking 'types' who I then would go on to fall into relationships with.

'Falling into their dick-sand' as Rebel Wilson said in that movie, How To Be Single.

I spent most of my adult life with a shovel, trying to dig myself out of that shit.

I'm sure men feel the same way sometimes:

Two drunks were sitting at a nightclub bar, and one said to the other, 'I'm so glad I turned to the bottle, instead of picking up these bloody women.'

'That's fine,' said the other drunk, 'Until you get your dick stuck!'

Drink chose all of my relationships, all of my life – and that's why until I got sober, none of them worked.

Because what Drinking Me thought was a fine match, Sober Me thought otherwise.

But because Drinking Me was the entity that my drinking man would be partnering, Sober Me didn't get a look in. And these men knew – and would *say* – that as long as they kept me drinking, everything was okay.

Sometimes, this remark would even be made about me in front of friends.

'Oh, yeah, we're doin' fine, so long as I keep her pissed!'

The bloke would laugh as he said it. I'd laugh too. And the friend – depending on if they were a real friend or not – would look either amused, or aghast.

But these guys knew to keep their fridges well-stocked for the next time I saw them – because I never would tolerate sober time with any of them.

Thus, the relationships would go on, until either the bloke couldn't stand my push and pull style any longer (I love you, now fuck off) – or Sober Me finally won out, and we got rid of him.

And then I'd go and drink and stumble my way into the next pile of dick-sand.

Doh.

But oh, I was so sick of partnering drunks, almost as much as I was sick of being one.

I attracted them like magnets.

At one stage, I even thought of posting a profile on one of those dating sites like Plenty of Fish, something along these lines:-

WANTED: I'm seeking a genuine addict who will promise to treat me badly, but also have the commitment to stick around forever, no matter what. Alcoholism, chain smoking, gambling, unsolicited sex & cheating, the more the better. These fine traits will make you financially irresponsible as well, and always broke, and I love that because I'm a hard worker, and I just live to prop up your lifestyle. No home, no problem —- I have a lovely home I'm working my guts out to pay off, and I really want to share it with you for free, so you can live here and control me - because that's what I need. A car and a licence isn't important, because I want a man I can drive around, especially to the bottle shop, and at least daily. I'd prefer also that you had no friends, and are willing to alienate mine, so we can be alone in our sick little love cocoon. If you're untrustworthy, lie and cheat, that's an added bonus because I love surprises, especially when your women knock on my door. Anger problems and violence are welcomed also; I just thrive on the drama, especially when it can be fuelled by alcohol or drugs, to add that element of real dangerousness to it, because I do so like to live on the edge. Your advanced stalking skills will also add to my experience, so don't be shy. Basically, if you can provide the rollercoaster, I'll ride it with you forever, because you're my man!

The real problem of course would be getting inundated.

Start as you intend to go on, a wise person once said.

If you want a relationship fuelled by alcohol (Sober Me didn't) then don't start that way.

So, whilst acknowledging that most sexual relationships would never even get off the ground without alcohol, deciding to be an undrinker in a drinking world also means choosing a partner that will sustain and nurture the Real You...

But if you're already in a relationship, in a threesome with you, your partner and the drink, basically when the drink goes, you've just got to assess what you're left with, and if it's salvageable. And it *will* be, so long as you're both on the same page about the departure of that third wheel.

Sadly, too many couples aren't.

I spent a long time, and quite a few relationships, with my own flawed way of thinking around drinking and dating, which went like this:

My drinking is only a problem when I'm in relationships – because when I'm single and drinking, I'm just a happy drunk that everybody likes. But when I'm drinking within relationships, I get sad and messy.

Hmm.

Therefore I can only conclude – that *relationships* are bad for me.

It's the relationship making me drink, and cry, and argue.

It didn't happen before the relationship came along.

Therefore – lose the relationship – but – *for fuck's sake, keep drinking!*

Phew.

Problem solved.

Till the next one.

You can see why I needed to write this book.

So I could keep it on my bookshelf for future reference.

7

Drinking and Parenting

'Being a parent drives me to drink,' is a pretty common motherism. And it doesn't seem to matter if you've got your gloriously nuclear family intact, or you're winging it solo, happily or unhappily. Parenting is hard work, most would agree.

Let's get into the two styles of parenting – they're pretty simple. Sober parenting. And drinking parenting. And how they differ.

I can definitely comment on this, because I've done both.

For much of my parenting experience, I was sober. All through my daughter's younger years, I was present, in every way a mother can be present for her child. Her life was tranquil, and safe, and she had certainty around her trust in me. I'd pick her up from school every day, and I'd be early.

I was present, to hear about her day, to help her with any problems, or her homework. Sometimes I even did it for her, especially if the project interested me. I remember when she was about seven years old, she (we) turned in a very cool assignment which featured a photo of my red V8 Ford at the time.

(The teacher was puzzled, but gave her three gold stars. A proud mum moment.)

I planned fun things for us to enjoy, with lots of good bonding time, and I opened our home to her friends in the same safe, loving way.

She tells me now, at the age of 23, that her childhood was as close to idyllic as it could be. And I'm going to go out on a limb here and say that my sobriety, and *presence* had a fair bit to do with that.

Because when drinking stepped into the picture, when she was around age 13, chaos entered the door at the same time - as well as unpresence, unlistening, and, well, lots of uns, for the first time. Because while I still *went through the motions* for her, and she got to school, with clean clothes, and had food to eat, et cetera – suddenly, I stopped making that best effort I always had. Because I simply wasn't always present, to be able to do so.

Drinking changed my priorities, and that changed the way I related to my daughter, and how much I was really, authentically present for her.

I found myself in a relationship with – as I said earlier – a good looking drinking bum of a man, who liked nothing better than providing me with beer, every day, straight into my own fridge, and staying every night at my place to enjoy said alcohol with me. He showed absolute disregard for my daughter's feelings, or our previously peaceful household – and I'm ashamed to say I completely enabled it!

I didn't want to give up the drinking, or the man, or the way those things made me feel when I was doing them. I felt like I was the queen of my own party. I suddenly had lots of drinking buddies, a partner to step out with, and a daughter who Drink had decided was old enough to pretty much fend for herself, both emotionally and physically.

I know this sounds awful, but it's what happened.

Sure, there was food in the fridge, and she wasn't in any actual danger (that I know of) – but I basically stopped taking the time to inquire into her world. To make sure she was doing okay. To see if she needed anything from me.

I became *un-present* as a parent. I see that now.

I wasn't always drunk, I might add. But as the drink slowly took a stranglehold on me, my head space became ever more consumed, not just with the drinking itself, but with thoughts of drinking – and looking forward to the next time I would drink – and then resenting the times I couldn't drink as much as I wanted.

The head space that drinking takes up is quite incredible. The planning, the purchasing, the socialising – and the recovery.

There were times I was simply too hungover to be present - so it wasn't just the drinking time – it was the hours, or even the full days I needed to recover. It was the way the whole practice of drinking slowly took over my life, like a cancer. And I just - couldn't - see it.

Wouldn't see it.

All I could see was that I deserved to have fun now, after being a single parent for so long, and I was damn well going to have that fun!

I never thought for a moment what example I was setting for my daughter, either. I didn't even know if she was drinking, herself. I didn't think to ask. Our communication, once so amazing, had gone down the S-bend. She now told me nothing. What's more - I didn't even *notice* she was telling me nothing!

I found out later that she'd been complaining about me to her dad – which enraged me – where it should have caused me to take a good hard look at myself. Because she had validity to her complaints. And when he started calling me a piss-head, I'd just about had enough - because by then, that label was becoming ingrained, from too many different people.

But I never questioned why this had happened to me. I just became angry, and resentful.

Eventually, my daughter decided that living with her dad was a better option – and Drinking Me said, 'Yep, fine, off you go then.' And then Sober Me felt like I'd had my heart torn out, having my daughter now living two states away, *and* no longer speaking to me. And I can tell you, no amount of alcohol, or fancy man, or drinking buddies, could soothe me at that point.

I ended up in counselling.

I also ended up single, because while I was ready to take responsibility for my behaviour, my big-drinking good-time man certainly wasn't up for that kind of accountability – and flatly denied the existence of any problems. As far as he was concerned, my daughter had left, he'd moved in immediately, and that *should* be enough for me.

It wasn't.

I now know – *the most important gift we ever give our children is our presence.* Our full, undivided attention, our teaching, and the gift of our life experience.

Drinking took me away from that state of giving. I could no longer prioritise my daughter's teen problems and development, alongside alcohol.

Alcohol takes much, and gives nothing.

It demands priority, and seeks to destroy anything in its path.

And the trouble is, in that struggle for my attention and my soul, alcohol put up a behemoth of a fight – and it won.

I didn't want my daughter to go. But Alcohol did. Alcohol knew I'd be able to drink *even more* if she went! And then, there'd be nothing left for me - except Alcohol.

From an unknown author: (paraphrased)

"Allow me to introduce myself. I am the disease of Alcohol – and I am cunning, baffling, and powerful.

That's Me. I have harmed millions, and I am pleased. I hate anyone with a solution, or a 'Higher Self.' To all who come in contact with me, I wish you suffering and I wish you death.

I love to catch you with the element of surprise. I love pretending I am your friend, and lover. I have given you comfort, haven't I? Wasn't I there when you were lonely? When you wanted to die, didn't you call on me? I WAS THERE!

I love to make you hurt. I love to make you cry. Better yet, I love to make you numb so you can neither hurt nor cry – when you can't feel anything at all. This is true gratification, and all I ask from you is long-term suffering. I've been there for you, always.

When things were going all right in your life, you invited me. You said you didn't deserve the good things, and I was the only one who would agree with you. Together, we were able to destroy all the good things in your life. People don't take me seriously. They take strokes, heart attacks, diabetes seriously – but not Me.

FOOLS! Without my help, none of this misery would be possible. I am such a hated disease, and yet I do not come uninvited. You choose to have me. Many have chosen me, over security and peace.

More than you hate me, I hate all of you who have a Higher Self. This weakens me, and I can't function in the manner I am accustomed to.

Now I must lie here quietly. You don't see me, but I am growing bigger and stronger than ever. When you only exist, I may live. When you live, I can only exist.

But I am here, until we meet again. If we meet again, I wish you suffering, denial, despair, anger, untruthfulness, and above all, DEATH.

THEN I'LL WIN."

#

And that, dear reader, is what Alcohol does best.

It destroys all that's precious around you. And at that point, it had done its job.

I felt obliterated.

Everything had been built on the illusion that is alcohol. The good-looking partner, the fun times on the drink – all disappeared like farts in the wind, once I brokenheartedly held up a mirror to myself.

Alcohol doesn't stick around for the hard stuff, the soul searching, the reflection.

It's a fucking fickle friend.

And it's a Lie.

But it so entrenches itself into your life; it gets into your brain and creates neural links all over the place, to every activity you ever enjoyed – until the idea of untangling from it appears too monstrously difficult to ever contemplate.

You feel as if there's no life without it. Or with it.

That is what Alcohol does.

8

Uncategorised Chaos

Of course, I don't wish to restrict the benevolence of our Social Substance – after all, it's a giving beast – and it has so much more misery to dish out yet.

These other concepts really warrant a chapter each, so great is the toll from them, but I'm writing a book here, not an encyclopedia.

Trust me when I say that by the time you finish this little tome, you'll know everything you need to know about alcoholic chaos, and I'm especially hoping there's some useful experience in here that you haven't considered thus far in your drinking career – and which might be the game changer for you. Because once you really see and understand what you're dealing with, and why, the way to fix it becomes far less complicated.

Are you ready?

I call this chapter Chaos, but it could also be unmitigated chaos. Let's start with risk-taking, because that often leads to the chaoses I'm going to cover here. Ooh, a new word. (Chaoi?) Yeah, let's do it that way – and pronounce it like kay-eye.

Chaos multiple. Indulge me. I love new words.

Risk-taking, ah.

Well, life's a risk, you say. You could get hit by a bus when you cross a road. Sure you can, except you know to look both ways first. But attempt to cross a busy road with a point two blood alcohol reading, and suddenly the odds of you stepping out in front of *any* vehicle, not just the cliched bus, increases exponentially.

So when I say risk-taking, I'm not referring to conscious risk-taking - those are merely the calculated chances we take every day - even just by getting out of bed in the morning without first checking the floor hasn't dropped away during the night.

We know the odds. It's pretty safe.

Unconscious risk-taking though is the sort of risk you'll take without a cognisant decision to do so.

Like going home with a stranger (who could turn out to be Ted Bundy's love child).

Like taking some weird homemade pill at a club, because everyone's raving about it – and winding up in the ER – or dead.

Like deciding to take an ocean swim at night, just because it's hot and you're on holiday (and pissed) – but there's an eager bull shark about three metres away from where you jumped in.

I still count myself lucky on a stinking hot day I got stuck out at Litchfield National Park Falls, that I'd had no alcohol with me, or in me. That wee little 'possible crocodiles in area' sign might not have deterred Drinking Me, desperate as I was to cool down and all.

Anyway, you get the picture.

Cognisant (thinking) risk-taking, as opposed to unconscious – and that's because the demon drink is holding your consciousness to ransom for the time being.

And it's dicing with death – yours - simply because that's what it loves to do!

Risk-taking via alcohol also has a part to play in just about every violent crime ever committed – and even some non-violent ones. Add in stupid crime as well.

Dumb ways to die (catchy little song - find it on YouTube).

From the big wannabe nightclub bouncer who decides to cave someone's head in merely for looking at them the wrong way (or not) – to the guy who decides, under the influence, to even give the bouncer that look in the first place. Or call him a few choice names. Whatever. Things nobody in their right mind would do – but somehow alcohol gives them the (soon to be crushed) nads/head/ego to do it.

The big kahuna of all alcohol-related violent crime of course is murder and manslaughter – and it's not a step too far along from other violent crime. Just taken to the next level. Not necessarily planned that way, mind you – but if your mind is bent out of shape by the 'social substance' – and you're fired by fury at the same time – well, nothing is off the cards, is it?

You're not thinking – you're angry – and there are no consequences because you're disinhibited.

Just for long enough, for the conditions to be right.

Rape and sexual assaults are great candidates for alcohol to play with also. I know even 40-odd years ago, some of the sex I had back then wasn't exactly 'consensual sex' – it was more like someone taking advantage of me because I was drunk. And me being silent on it afterwards, of course.

Embarrassed.

Mortified. And resolving to do better next time.

Just not drink less, the one thing that would've kept me safe.

These days, of course, more of these kinds of incidents end up as charged acts in the County Court, and rightfully so. And nowhere is the 'pissed elephant in the room' syndrome quite as alive as in our justice system.

Because while drinking is acknowledged as at least part of the problem, in no way does anybody ever suggest that young girls wouldn't be in this situation if they abstained from drinking alcohol. It's just treated as an accepted fact that young people drink too much, and that sometimes if they're unlucky, it leads to this kind of offending.

Ditto for the young men involved, who might sheepishly feel that the girl was willing (perhaps because she was unconsciously drunk, and therefore not actively refusing) and so it was, at worst, an *error of judgment*. Because, hey, he was pissed too.

And if at the end of it you merely ended up with an unwanted pregnancy, or an STD – I guess that's still a minor league outcome, when you consider what could have been.

Often, of course, the drinking victim is grilled in the witness box far more vigorously on account of her lack of control around her drinking, than the perpetrator is regarding his choice to commit a sex crime. And his drinking?

Meh.

Boys will be boys, right?

I'll repeat again – *none of these "misunderstandings" happen between sober people!*

Gambling is another biggie.

The hotels of course have their quota of poker machines, adjacent to their bars – and encourage their patrons to freely partake of both. After all, it's a free country, and if you lose all your money while getting pissed at the pokies, it's *your* fault for not having the control to know when to stop.

Easy cop out.

The gambler goes home with an empty bank account, and wonders how it happened, and worse, how they're going to tell their partner all that money's gone. It's much easier to lie about that too!

Ditto the guy at the TAB, betting on the horses. Not only is his judgment impaired from the alcohol, and the odds are stacked against him making an intelligent choice – but again the bar is conveniently at hand to drown his sorrows afterwards, or keep him betting until he's out of loot.

See the connection yet?

Do you think it's by accident – or by design?

And who stands to benefit from it, aside from the hotelier and the brewers, if it is in fact 'by design'?

More on that later.

Then you've got the unfortunate souls who end up jobless and destitute, on account of their drinking - and let's not forget the rampant absenteeism that goes with alcoholism.

It matters not, because the drink will step in (for the drinker) when things go pear-shaped, to numb the damage in the moment – and ensure the poor sod has no way out of his predicament. Because instead of taking a forthright approach, with admissions of poor judgment (which might have saved his career) what does he do?

Bingo.

He drinks *more*. And kills off any possibility of redemption.

Now he's facing financial ruin, marriage breakdown and the like.

What does he do about that then?

Yep.

You got it – he drinks *even more*.

Drink driving is another goodie. If you've got a bit of age on you – I have, but I like to call it worldly wisdom, ha – you'll remember a time when drink driving was a common thing. It certainly predated booze buses and breathalysers.

It wasn't even shameful; you just did it. After all, you had to get home, right?

Back in the day, we'd all pile in the car together, with no thought of how drunk the driver might be. If they could hold the steering wheel and sit upright, and coordinate forward momentum on the pedals, we were good to go! And that was minus seat belts.

These days of course, with the rise of drink-driving offences, this simply highlights the problem that is alcohol. Judgment and drinking don't generally co-exist well together.

They never did.

You might feel that just because things are a bit blurry, you'll be okay. Because who knows what .05 feels like anyway, or how different it is for each individual?

So, risks are taken.

Sometimes they're catastrophic, for you, or for some random innocent party whose path you might cross at that time. Or sometimes they're just deadly to your career, or your family.

Even if you've only had one or two drinks, we all know that

sense of your heart skipping a beat, and that cold dread of fear, upon rounding a corner and seeing those blue and red flashing lights, and the burly policeman standing in the middle of the road, waving you in for a breath test.

And if you do get caught being over the legal limit - but keep on drinking because you find you can't stop - your life then becomes a revolving door of court appearances, loss of licence, alcohol re-education classes - or perhaps the ultimate humiliation of having a device fitted to your car that won't allow you to drive until you blow a zero reading into it.

And paying stacks of money to the government for the privilege – for years.

Needless to say, you'll never experience, or even have to think about, any of these issues as a non-drinker.

It's bloody liberating.

A chapter like this wouldn't be complete without the mother of all crime, and that one belongs to suicide.

Suicide is a crime against Self, and against Soul. And it's fitting that alcohol nearly always plays a part in suicide attempts – because alcoholism is a self-inflicted crime against Self.

It's a natural, convenient stepping stone.

Suicide is never a step people take when they're in their Higher Selves. And alcohol is a certain way to tip you into your lower self, every single time.

It numbs you, and it magnifies your problems – without ever offering any hope of solutions. Your only solution is to numb it more, by drinking more.

It's a progressive fall from grace, and hope.

That's what alcohol offers you.

It's *all* it offers you.
And to my mind, that's no offer at all.

9

How Do I Stop?

Great info – BUT HOW DO I STOP?

I'd like to say it's simple – and the solution really *is* simple. But the process isn't. And what's more, it's different for every drinker.

But first and foremost, the toughest, most stubborn hurdle will be ... DENIAL.

Denial that you've got a problem.

Even when consciously you know, and admit, that drinking is causing big problems for you - your subconscious will be in denial, just so it can keep you stuck drinking. And denial will arise under all sorts of auspices. You need to watch out for them.

Here's a few to get you started:

I haven't got a drinking problem because:

I don't drink every day.

I don't start drinking before 5 pm.

I only drink on the weekends.

I'm a *fun* drinker.

People prefer me when I'm drinking, so how can that be a

problem?

Everybody tells me I don't have a drinking problem.

I can stop at one or two.

I can stop anytime.

(Try it)

There's no alcoholism in my family (I heard this one from a lady who would drink a bottle of wine a night – but it was *only* one bottle, she said.)

I only drink when I'm out.

I only drink when I'm at home.

I drink because I'm alone and sad, and it's not hurting anyone (else.)

I only drink when I'm stressed.

I drink because of the way my family treats me, or my friends, or the guy at the corner store, or my boss.

I'm not an alcoholic, because my alcohol counsellor said I'm only alcohol dependent.

(Er – what's the difference?)

I drink because the world has gone mad.

(Tip: it has, and for everybody)

If I could get a job, I'd stop drinking.

If I could lose weight, I'd be happier and stop drinking.

If only I didn't have financial problems

(Tip: those will get worse)

You'll come up with a million reasons for your drinking, and why it *isn't* a problem.

And yet – you're reading this book.

Right?

So there's a concerned inner Self, buried deep in you, that really, really doesn't want to keep doing this to yourself. It wants to find answers.

You're hoping of course for an easy fix – and there isn't any.

You've got to do the work.

So, here's the first bit. This got me on my way to sobriety, back in 2019, after yet another unplanned bender left me bereft and sobbing on my bed, and knowing – *knowing*, I could not keep going on this way.

Go get a big piece of paper, blank on both sides. And a pen.

Yes, you know what's coming – and I promise you, it's the beginning of a game-changer.

I'll wait.

#

Welcome back.

This is going to sound familiar – from my own awakening process – but here I am, offering the same humble beginnings, to you.

You're going to make two lists.

That's all I'm going to ask of you today.

Two lists.

Let's do the first one, first.

I'm a methodical chick.

I want you to write down every reason you can think of, for why you drink. No matter how poignant, how tiny, how embarrassing, how anything.

Just get them all out.

This is just for you – you don't ever need to show this list to anybody!

And while you do this, I'll share what a few of mine were back in 2019.

My reasons for drinking: (clears throat) –
   Because I'm stressed about being in a relationship.
   Because I need the confidence when running events (I was a social club organiser).
   Because I'd be boring without it.
   I like the taste of beer on a hot day.
   It's a social thing to do.
   People like me as a drinker (and tell me so!)
   I'd never be able to have sex, or be in a relationship, without it.
   It's such a huge part of my life, I can't imagine not drinking.
   It relaxes me.
   It helps me sleep at night.

I could go on – but those were the ones off the top of my head, back then.

How's your list going? Do you have lots of reasons?

#

Now – List No.2 – *listen up* –
   Turn your trusty piece of paper over – and I now want you to write the reasons you *no longer* wish to drink.
   Just list them.
   This is about what drinking *doesn't* do for you – or the problems it causes for you.
   It can be anything.
   But you want to stop (or drink less) because of ….

(And here's mine, again off the top of my head from 2019):

My drinking worries me, as it gets out of control.

I have no off button when I drink.

I have no filters when I drink.

It stresses me how much money I'm spending on drinking.

I'm scared for my health.

Some days my head is so sore I feel like I'm dying. I'm killing myself.

I worry about what I do and say when intoxicated.

I worry about the name I am getting around town, as a piss-head.

I'm tired of losing things like my phone, or my wallet (or my mind!) when I'm drunk.

I get scared of the risks I take when drunk, like walking home alone at 2 am.

I keep finding myself in crappy relationships with drinkers, and then expend a lot of energy trying to get out of them – and then I drink more because it's too hard.

I'm tired of losing so much of my time to drinking, and recovering from drinking.

I feel nothing will ever change for me while I'm a drinker.

I will never meet authentic friends while I'm a drinker.

I'll never meet a decent partner as a drinker.

I don't like a lot of the people I hang out with as a drinker.

I hate myself for being unable to function socially without a drink in my hand.

I can't sleep properly anymore, and so I'm developing a reliance on sleeping pills.

I'm sad most of the time when I'm sober, and all I think about is my next drinking session. I'm wishing my life away.

#

Phew.

Did you come up with a few?

For me, it was a trip down memory lane – but it's now a gratitude exercise, when I look at these lists today. I realise that whole mindset has now gone – and I'm so *grateful* it makes me tear up.

Back to you.

If you've exhausted your two lists, you've probably got a lot of stuff whirling around in your head right now. Because it's incredible when we really sit down, and honestly appraise the situation. Not in front of anyone, so there's no excuses that need to be made.

Just you, sitting there, with your wee little pen and big sheet of paper, now covered in writing.

Have a re-read of what you've written, and add in any more you might have missed.

No rush.

#

The next bit is the fun part – well, insofar as any of this can be fun – but I'll try and keep it light-hearted for you. Because this exercise brought me realisations which truly blew my mind.

Most importantly, it opened my mind to the idea of finally, truly questioning *what drinking actually did for me.*

So, now - I want you to match up your reasons FOR drinking, and NOT drinking.

Huh?

Yep.

I'm not saying *all* the reasons we drink are contradictions – but a fair few of them will be. And this exercise illustrates, better than any other I've seen, the contradiction that is alcohol.

How it actually *creates* the problems for us, to then give us *reasons* for the drinking.

Okay, let me illustrate a couple of mine to get you started – or you can even play around with mine to begin with, if you like!

I drink to be social – vs – I worry about how I've treated people when I'm drunk.

My drinking relaxes me - vs - I'm stressed because my drinking gets out of control.

People like me as a drinker - vs - I don't even like half the people I hang out with / I'll never find real and authentic friends while I drink.

I'll never be able to have sex, or be in a relationship without drinking - vs - I keep finding myself in crappy relationships with drinkers, and then spending all my time trying to get out of them.

So, just to take those first few examples above, let me paraphrase it.

I drink to be social, but my social drinking self is out of control. I go around offending people because I have no filters when drunk, and I'm also getting a bad name around town. All in the name of drinking to be social.

(Doesn't sound too smart)

And my drinking relaxes me, but when I'm sober I feel *stressed* about my drinking, and how long it takes to recover from my drinking, and what it's doing to my health, and my friendships, and just my life in general.

(Doesn't sound too relaxing)

People like me as a drinker, but I don't even like some of these people I drink with. In fact, I wish I could meet new friends where I didn't have to drink just to be around them.

(Sounds like I'm drinking *for* those people, and not for me)

I'll never be able to have sex or relationships without drinking, but I hate the relationships I end up in, so much so that I escalate my drinking to escape my feelings around them.

(Alcohol chooses my relationships – and it's not discerning – so I have to drink more alcohol to sustain being in those relationships)

#

I've just used those four examples to illustrate my own contradictory beliefs around alcohol - and how following this little exercise through, I reached conclusions which flew in the face of my reasons for drinking in the first place.

Drinking suddenly made no sense at all to me, once I saw this.

If you can reach some of your own conclusions by doing this exercise, that's the goal here. And I have to warn you, it's not for the faint hearted.

You'll discover things about yourself, and your drinking, that you really don't like. And yet you're not *really* discovering some of them for the first time, are you? Because deep down, you've known the drink is creating lots of un-good feelings and actions for you.

But laying them out bare like this, to see them clearly, is confronting – and yet it's so liberating too!

If you have a very trusted and supportive friend, you could show them what you've written. I didn't. I was too embarrassed.

But now here I am, putting it in a book for the whole world to see!

Being able to share could at least open up a dialogue with a friend.

It takes the problem out of isolation.

Unfortunately for me though, by this time I was just too ashamed of myself, and had kept the extent of the problems my drinking had created for me largely hidden.

I'd lived an illusion for a long time, you see.

Truth doesn't sit well with alcohol abuse.

It's often why we drink in the first place, to not have to face it.

#

The reason this little exercise is so powerful is because it addresses the problem where it really starts – and ends. Which is in the drinker's brain.

I call it Drinking Brain.

Drinking Brain gave you all the reasons you love to drink.

And then Sober Brain provided you with all of the reasons you don't want to drink like that anymore.

These two parts of your brain are currently in conflict. And we've all heard of cognisant dissonance, right? It's been in the media for lots of reasons of late. But in case you haven't, cognisant dissonance occurs when the higher side of your brain (in this case Sober Brain) gets overridden by the lower side of your brain (Drinking Brain) even though *you know* Sober Brain is inherently correct, and has your best interests. And because you can't understand why you're listening to Drinking Brain when you *know* Sober Brain is right, it creates a tear in your psychic fabric, if you like – or a split.

That split enables you to compartmentalise those two conflicting views you hold, so that you can then hold them *both*, within the same brain, and at the same time. Which means you can, and will, continue to do what you *know* isn't serving you.

It's effectively ignoring your Higher Self, that part of you that only wants the best for you.

The same thing occurs in an abusive relationship, where the abused partner continues to remain in it. You can bet they know why they *shouldn't* be there, but they somehow override their better self to remain in it, sometimes until they get killed.

It is this rupture in your thinking that keeps you doing or believing something, when your own self knows it's detrimental to continue doing that.

By compartmentalising it, it's like hiding the lie from the truth.

The dark from the light.

Except you're not really hiding it, just obfuscating it, in this case, by getting numb by drinking.

Because knowing your truth sometimes feels unbearably painful.

Drinking serves a lot of purposes in this regard, by its numbing qualities alone.

People want relief.

They want that quick fix. And drinking pretends to offer that.

Because not only does it numb away your problems – only temporarily, mind – but it also gives you a shot of *high* while doing so. Temporary also. And that high becomes more fleeting, the more you go on.

So you have to drink *more*, and drink it *more quickly*. Otherwise the high dissipates, and the downer quickly follows.

No drinker ever enjoys coming down.

Drinking is also a depressant – and by engaging in the substance regularly, you will end up depressed and anxious, and feeling hopeless and out of control.

No problems ever got faced and solved while on the drink, even though it's joked about between drinkers that no problem is ever so big that a drink can't fix it.

You're kidding yourself.

But you already know that.

#

But I love the taste...

This is the one drinking reason you'll come up with that you won't necessarily have a direct contradictor for. And I can guarantee that just about *every* drinker will have this on their reasons to drink list, and probably quite high up on it.

I know I did.

So this one deserves a little para of its own – because I just happen to have a contradictor for this one also!

(Drum roll)

Deciding you enjoy the taste of alcohol is just a *learned behaviour*.

Think back to the first time ever that you drank.

It might have been a little bit of wine that your parents offered you as a kid. Or it might have been a beer at a party, or some shots.

But the first time you taste that stuff – it's got bones in it, man.

It tastes shit – because it *is* shit.

It's what they make car fuel out of. Ethanol. Not good for humans.

Poison.

And your body rejected it, the first time you drank too much – and that's because the body rejects poisons, in order to survive. It gets you to throw up the offending substance.

But wait, you say. My first drink was a Cruiser, or a UDL, and it tasted just like soft drink. Or a pear cider – that tasted great, and it's probably even kind of healthier, right? Or I had a rum and coke – and yeah, okay, it made the coke taste not quite as nice – but I won't say I *hated* it. So, there.

Listen up.

What you 'enjoyed' in any, or all of the above drinks, my drinking friend, was *not* the alcohol.

It was the *sugar added to the alcohol.*

Sugar being another addiction, of course. And it's no surprise there are now so many sugared, alcoholic drinks out there, for the kids to ease their way into the drinking trap.

Heck, they even put sugary substances into vapes, the latest deadly craze to hit the human race. And guess what?

The kids are hooked.

Just like that.

Worse than cigarettes.

Cigarettes never smelt, nor tasted so good. How could something that tastes, or smells, so innocently *sweet* – be dangerous?

Well – it's deadly dangerous.

So, basically, if you say you love the taste of alcohol – you either love the *effects* of it so much that you've grown a tolerance, and possibly a liking over time, for the taste of it – or you love the sugar in it, which makes it easier to access said effects.

Or you might have another reason you say you love it. You might be convinced it *goes well* with an Italian meal, or fine dining.

As if nothing else could do the trick!

Rest assured though – what you're drinking it for is the *effect*.

Because if it had no effects at all (such as a chocolate milkshake) you'd maybe have one occasionally, but you wouldn't suddenly lose control over your intake one day, and regrettably stuff down eight of them, before you knew it was happening. Or drink a couple every night when you're home alone, just because they go well with something you're eating.

I should mention also the psychological aspects of why you might believe you like the substance. Isn't it also the fitting in, perhaps with a certain demographic – or even possibly a group you might aspire to belong to? That it actually can appear to be grown-up, glamorous even, to wrap your long red manicured fingernails around what you're assured is a *quality* glass of fine red?

(Note: it's been shown that after a few drinks, even 'fine wine connoisseurs' radars tend to go down the S-bend when it comes to discerning what it is they're actually ingesting. Yet another lie.)

You don't love the taste of alcohol.

Alcohol itself is a poison, and poison doesn't taste good.

You've developed a *liking* for your hybrid, mass-marketed substance, but it's because you *love its effects* – or you *need* its effects.

Let that really, really sink in.

And if you don't believe me – go and taste some *pure* alcohol – no additives - not too much, we don't want to kill you! – and then come back here and tell me how great it tasted.

#

So, to recap –

Alcohol is not your friend.

Alcohol, in and of itself, tastes like a toxic chemical.

It's a legitimate poison.

And yet half the world is addicted to it – and many are in denial about their use of it.

Remember, people are addicted to things like paint and glue sniffing, heroin, cocaine, vaping – and they're all chasing the same thing.

A feeling that's *different* to who they naturally, organically *are*.

The fact that some choices are legitimised and some aren't is really inconsequential. They're still all addictive substances.

So it's time to ask yourself – if it's not serving your interests to be addicted to this substance, well, then – who is it serving?

Alcohol and your government.

Interesting title, that – and when I say 'your government' I don't necessarily mean the parliamentarians running the circus – I'm talking about *your* government, i.e. the government, or *governing* of YOU, the individual:

How do you govern masses and masses of people with differing ideas?

What common denominator could the masses be governed with?

Is there a legal substance that we can socially encourage, to do the heavy lifting for us?

Alcohol is the ultimate weapon of governments.

Think about it.

People who are sold with the idea of numbing themselves, whether for fun, or to numb pain, or hopelessness, or loneliness, or a million other reasons that will never be solved by drinking – will only know *one reaction* to any further challenge life throws at them.

And that's to drink again – or drink more.

Governments know this.

And having now enabled much of the population to partake of the 'essential service that is alcohol' *as much as they wanted*, during the recent lengthy lockdowns, it's unsurprising that so many more people now have serious drinking problems than they did prior. And because they've now been subconsciously encouraged to turn to alcohol at a time they felt powerless, it's now an *unconscious*, short step for them to continue to do so.

You weren't allowed to breathe fresh air, remember.

You weren't supposed to make a decision on your own bodily autonomy either.

But you could always drink.

During the lockdowns, things like gyms, or swimming pools, or even sitting on a blanket having a picnic with friends, or going to the beach, were outlawed as 'too risky.' You couldn't get a haircut - unless you were a politician's wife. And hefty fines were dished out for daring to flout the government rules that were put there to 'keep everybody safe.'

But heck – get over to your local bottle-o and pick yourself up a few slabs – or better still, home delivery - *drink till you die* in the permitted space of your own home – there's nothing risky about *that*, right?

You'll need it, to cope with your kids being cooped up in there with you, month after month – because playgrounds have been outlawed, alongside schools, alongside many people's livelihood.

Just not alcohol.

Never alcohol - the essential service, granted to all. And in some cases, with government handouts to finance it.

(I'm not saying all people went down this path, by the way. Some enlightened souls really used the 'slow time' to connect with themselves, to wind back the pace of life, and to disconnect from the hustle culture. To really start viewing the world with a clear lens. Adversity brings out the most amazing things in people, when alcohol isn't numbing what we're all truly capable of.)

But the fallout from this pandemic period is immense, and ongoing. For one thing, many people are more anxious, more depressed, more isolated.

They'd had to tolerate being locked down – curfewed even - and without ever a lock. And subjected to conditions out of their control – they turned to the one thing that blotted it all out for them.

Alcohol.

Nice, legal alcohol, *always* available, with stamp of approval from your caring government.

The elephant in the room is WHY.

I'll tell you why.

It's in the interests of governments to keep the masses unthinking, dumbed down, and drunk. The more willing, the better.

Alcohol equals inertia.

Not only can heavy drinkers not solve their own problems, they aren't ever going to take on the real issues in the world, beginning with what's going on at the top. And our conditioning keeps us exactly where they want us.

At the bottle shop hypermart, with a trolley, credit card in hand.

Decades ago, in Russia, alcohol was readily available, and cheaper than a loaf of bread – so desirable was it that the masses keep drinking. I wouldn't say it's like that in Australia – except it kind of is.

Of course, the more 'discerning' drinker won't be satisfied with a bottle of Passion Pop at $4 a throw (less than your average loaf of bread, by the way) or crappy cask wine at $10 for four litres (about the same price as diesel, funny that!) But cheap piss has always been there for the taking, if and when the unfortunate drinker falls into financial crisis.

It's a bit like cigarettes years ago. In good times, people would choose Benson & Hedges for its gold packaging and illusion of wealth, or Marlborough for its rough and tough image. But when the financial shit hit the fan, brands like Longreach, which did huge packs for half the price and which I'm told tasted like camel dung heated up, were a sell-out sensation.

Now, of course, they can sell them wrapped in graphic

pictures illustrating what these chemical darts really do to your body. They could present them neatly wrapped in paperbark and dog turds for that matter - but people are addicted so as to turn a blind eye to all of that – *and* pay roughly ten times the amount they used to.

Such is the price of addiction.

The government call the shots – and when they need more income, they further tax the addicts.

And alcohol is absolutely no different.

Because once you're hooked, you're hooked.

You *need* your fix.

And that's pretty much all you're going to worry about, even with the world imploding around your ears.

Alcohol misuse also feeds entire industries – many of which are governmental – such as the health and medical industry.

Whether we're talking here about pharmaceutical sales, mental health services, doctors and clinics, counselling, social work, hospitalisation for alcohol related illnesses and accidents, rehab centres, dependency clinics – these industries would not be doing their roaring trade without alcohol feeding the problem.

But the news is curiously silent on suicide – there's no money to be made from that.

The dead don't spend.

Most of the health problem solutions offered are dependent on someone else fixing the drinker's problems – taking the responsibility, and ultimately the power, off of the drinker. Meaning that when the drinker relapses, as they assuredly will because they have handed over the problem to be solved by somebody else (and therefore the solution) - these institutions will be waiting with open arms to welcome them back for yet more *treatment.*

And then there's the media who are the governmental pimps – selling the dream to the masses, along with enough gaslighting to blow us all to the moon, drink firmly in hand, naturally.

I'm not going to harp on about this – it's not why I'm writing this book – but it's an important slice of the pie it would be remiss of me to omit.

Plus it addresses that old chestnut of 'If alcohol is so bad, why is it legal?'

Alcohol is the only legal substance that any adult can buy, that can dumb you down to the point of inaction in all areas of your life – and, more importantly, *keeps you there*!

And *that's* why it's there.

That's why it's *always* going to be there.

In our world.

And in your life, fuelling your own set of problems, and inertia to do anything about them.

Until you decide otherwise.

That's why it's marketed so vigorously.

That's why it's ever-present alongside gambling venues, sports events and the like.

It follows where the money runs, you see.

That's why it's made ever more attractive to young people (get 'em hooked early, for fuck's sake) – and that's why, in my view, the *only way* out of this bear trap is firstly understanding exactly what's going on here, with no filters, seeing it for what it is, and then deciding Hell No, you're done with it.

Make that done and a half!

We won't change governments anytime soon – the parties are merely different sides of the same beast.
But we can bloody well change ourselves.
Our power rests with us.
It's time to flex it.
Are you ready?

10

But Can I Moderate (Or Not)?

This idea, quite frankly, is a carrot that we as drinkers dangle in front of ourselves.

Because we don't want to actually 'give up' drinking (more on this later) – and all we really want is to be like all those other drinkers we know. You know, the ones that go out and have a good time without getting messy. Not that you really *notice* if they do or not, because when you're having that whale of a time yourself, you don't tend to notice much about anybody else.

You're numb, remember, even when that pretends to feel good. And your observations just aren't there.

Drink doesn't connect people – it's the polar opposite.

And then there's the majority of problem drinkers, and they're the ones who say they can 'take it or leave it', meanwhile sucking down a bottle of wine each night. But, hey, *they* don't have a problem.

You only have a problem if you see it, and then have the balls to actually admit it to yourself, never mind to others. So, sadly, we are in a minority.

Did I say earlier that alcoholism is *not* an honest addiction?

I'll say it again then.

Alcohol is a lie.

And it keeps us stuck in lies, in order to keep perpetuating it.

But let's get to Moderation, that holy grail of drinking. The thing most drinkers tell you they do with ease, and the rest of us shamefully strive for, and wonder why we can't.

I had my own attempts at moderation, and let me tell you, I'm pretty creative when I want something badly enough. And I really, really did not want to stop drinking.

At least, Drinking Brain really, really didn't want to. And that was the brain I listened to the most, for decades.

My own attempts at moderation began with things like Dry July, and Ocsober. Those forays into soberdom were mostly about reassuring myself that I really didn't have a problem, that I wasn't a (shudder) alcoholic – and the reason I would know this is by completing a month off the substance.

You see, I believed, along with most of the planet, that if you could stop for a month, you *obviously* didn't have a drinking problem.

Phew.

Here's a Facebook post of mine, dated 1 July 2011:

Me: Dry July – here I go!

Julie: Good luck, Caz.

Me: Thanks, Julie. Won't be easy but will try. At least it's not beer weather, hehehe.

Didi: You crazy lady, don't do it!!!

Me: Don't worry, I'm unlikely to succeed... Just thought I'd try it so I can confirm I'm an alcoholic! (winky face).

On 5 July, four days later, I updated my Facebook, posting that I'd already failed.
Responses:
Rosie: Hahaha – I also contemplated this and tried for one day... then I forgot why.
Didi: Doesn't prove you're an alcoholic, it proves you're normal!!
Oh my.

And then this, from my Ocsober 2013 blog:
"I emerge out of the surf, and stand there in the breeze, getting air dried. The guys with the beers are gone, thankfully. I start to walk along the sand. I can hear music coming from the surf club, so I want to get closer to hear what's playing. And of course, the first thing I notice is all the people on the deck, drinking, laughing and enjoying. I turn away, rinse my feet, then walk back towards the road. Past Laguna Jack's (and that bottle shop again) only this time there's a heap of people on Laguna's balcony, enjoying their icy cold bevies at this time of day. I grit my teeth. I now want one so bad, I almost consider cheating. I can feel my legs wanting to walk in there, to that big inviting glass fridge, choosing my preferred icy friend, cracking him and taking that first gulp, my fingers wet with cold moisture off the glass – and how great that would taste.

But then how bloody awful I'll feel, how I'll kick myself, how ashamed, how everything is BAD BAD BAD. Four days and couldn't cut it. And the alarming implications that raises in me, the suggestion that really I am no longer in control of my choices, because I need that drink more than I need to keep my integrity."

As you can see, it was no picnic.

And back then, I was really only what you'd call a 'weekend drinker.'

I went into Ocsober, proclaiming to everybody what I was doing, expecting it to be a bit irritating, but really I presumed I'd breeze through it. A month is only four weekends, after all.

But as you can see, it wasn't quite that easy.

(I didn't succeed either – I bought a house which settled on the 16th of the month, and how could you *not* have a beer to celebrate that!)

So it was just 15 days of sobriety for me – and I thankfully released that crazy idea, returning to my weekend binge drinking. Being "normal."

And the earlier Dry July effort never even got off the ground – how could it, with the kind of attitude I took into it?

The fact I was attempting it at all merely tells me I knew I had a problem, but was posting on Facebook to take the piss out of it, no pun intended.

Maybe I did it for Facebook likes – another fail, because there weren't any!

I then went on to try different means of moderation.

The first attempt, an obvious one, was to substitute full strength beer for light beer. Which tasted like shit, I thought. Well, all beer tastes like shit really, it's just that you want the maximum buzz as payoff for bulk-drinking a shit-tasting substance. Why ingest that crap and only get a quarter of the buzz? I'd have to drink four times the quantity. Eww.

As you can see from my mindset, that didn't even get off the ground. I tried it. I invested in one slab of lights, drank a couple – and then went out and bought a 'real' slab instead. The light fellas stayed in the fridge, to be inflicted upon visitors. It made me look benevolent because if they were driving, it meant I was looking out for them. They'd have the lights, and I'd be on the real stuff.

I might add, it took ages to get rid of those light suckers because not too many of my drinking visitors wanted them either!

I tried this a couple of times (just to be sure, to be sure) and it never worked. I just ended up with heaps of light beer, which I stored in the garage as it took up valuable fridge space.

And then I thought, well, if I don't like light, going *mid* is at least a step in the right direction - so I tried that for a time. And look, that went a little better, and by that I mean I didn't fail immediately. I lasted a little while – perhaps a month. I don't remember the time frame.

What I *do* remember clearly though was that while I was drinking mids, I *always* wanted full strength. Without exception. The mids tasted acceptable to me, sort of like the real thing – and probably did taste like the real thing – poison - but because I was aware of the numbers, psychologically I knew the buzz wouldn't be as strong. And instead of embracing that as a good thing, I just felt deprived. Peeved.

I guess I should, for completeness, mention zero-strength alcohol here – and yes, I tried that too – and that lasted exactly half of one beer. Sadly, I'd purchased six, so it was an expensive half can of toxic waste.

And I couldn't even give those suckers away.

#

And now for some Reverse Moderation Examples:

(Unsurprisingly, I was great at this!)

By the way, I was considering creating an Excesses chapter, but I realised pretty quickly that it would have swamped this book, while serving no useful purpose.

These are just a bit of light relief - but with a serious side, to illustrate how bad things got for me.

Cruise ship drinking stories - aha.

My partner, Michael, and I were on our first P&O cruise together, where our heavy drinking was off the Richter scale – and we were taking turns going up to the bar to buy rounds. I was on Carlton Draughts, and he wanted Great Northerns. But the only Northerns at this bar were mid strength.

So I came back with that first round of one Northern and one Carlton. Then he bought the next round, and so on and so forth.

He didn't realise until about the sixth round that he'd been drinking mids – and boy, was he pissed off about it! He immediately went into rectification mode – something only drinkers will understand – and not only upped the size of each drink to a pint of full strength, but he also managed a whole bottle of wine afterwards to, as he said, catch up!

Another typical story, this one courtesy of the beautiful Sun Princess Fijian cruise.

It's Australia Day 2019.

I'm about to order a cocktail (because after several days I'd grown sick of so much beer) when the barman informs us that Carlton Draughts are two pints for one, because of this oh-so-special drinking day.

My eyeballs, which had been scanning the cocktail menu, snapped around at those words, and immediately Drinking

Brain's accountant was madly calculating we could get pissed at an enormously reduced rate, if we could only cooperate together on this mission.

Of course, we did.

Six rounds of pints of full strength – that's over three litres of heavy beer for the uninformed – and I was ready to enter a pie eating competition, something that Drinking Brain decreed I'd *always* wanted to do.

Clearly it was a life mission, a calling, that Sober Brain wasn't aware of.

But - nobody else wanted to join in, and I needed competitors. I went around and muscled (bullied) a crew of warlike women to eat pies against, and after requesting big splatters of tomato sauce all round, we were off n' chomping!

I might add, just for context, those pies were big, with enormously thick crusts, and as dry as funeral scones. They were the most unpalatable pies you could imagine, like they'd been sitting in the crematorium below deck for the last 8 cruises, and now here was an opportunity to unload them onto a pack of piss-heads, with the promise of a bottle of champers for the wildebeest that could ingest them the fastest.

All this in the name of entertainment.

There were four pies each.

Just as we started, I asked Michael to fetch me another pint of draught, to help slide those pies down – which he duly obliged.

By the time he arrived back with it, I was on my second pie. I hadn't even managed to finish the first one in totality, as the crusts were so unforgiving – but I figured I'd get back to them later if there was time. I wasn't sure there would be, it was such a monster task.

I couldn't look at the other competitors – I was focused on

the job in front of me.

I found it best to just rest the pie on my lower jaw and just keep on snapping at it, like an anaconda consuming a deer. But I was just beginning on my third pie when the winner was announced.

I looked up incredulously, lips still wrapped around that parched pastry, and was sickened to see that indeed I was not the Pie Eating Champ of the Cruise, and never really had a hope.

Michael had taken a video of all that fun, and to this day I am mortified by what I saw.

I really did look like an anaconda consuming a pig. My chins looked about three times the size, so bloated were they with pastry – and I literally felt nauseated watching myself – and still do.

But I had managed about the same amount as my competitors – barring the winning warthog. She was the equivalent of a front-end loader, and had the process down pat, never faltering. She wasn't even an enormous lady – she just wanted that free bottle of plonk, she said!

I remember we congratulated her at the finish, and I'm looking at her belly, feeling so nauseated myself, and picturing those four pies nestled smugly in her guts. Mine by that stage were jostling uneasily in my stomach, amid the three litres of lager.

Not a nice sensation.

I might add, that night I was afraid they were going to have to airlift me off the ship as a medical emergency. The pain in my gut was intense.

(I'd been hospitalised about six months prior with a tear in the colon – poor toileting habits exacerbated by – you guessed it – drinking – and although I'd healed up, the pain still niggled at times to remind me when I overdid it.)

This pie-gobbling fun was way more than overdone – and again I berated myself for the abject stupidity of putting myself through something like this, given the frailty that still existed in my digestive system.

Alcohol is an inflammatory too, remember, and I just hadn't given it more than a week's rest since the hospital scare.

A week or so later, I read an article about a woman of around my age, on another cruise ship, who died after entering a lamington-eating competition that same Australia Day.

Poor lady.

Back to the ship.

Same day.

Michael, not to be outdone, had entered the sack race.

Now, this lovely fellow is unco at the best of times; he is 6 foot 2 of arms and legs, and can be clumsy sober.

The boys climbed into their sacks, and off they bounced. Michael took two enthusiastic leaps, and then fell over flat on his face. I filmed it, of course, though it was never going to compete with the pie-eating vid in our Hall of Shame. Luckily in the moment he wasn't hurt, just peeved at his lack of performance.

So, to rub it in, I decided to perform what I considered a graceful swan dive into the shallow end of the pool, just as I heard one of the staff call out, 'No, no, shallow end! Shallow end!'

Too late.

I was midair, my arms came out, and on that day I realised, if I hadn't before, that there was a God, and He was looking out for me.

I felt my belly graze the bottom of the pool as I came in on just enough angle not to break my neck.

I resolved not to drink like that again on Australia Day.

And still on that same ship - we'd arrived at the beautiful island of Lifou for a day off the ship. A rest from the drinking perhaps.

I'd taken some space for myself, to explore the island on my own.

But Michael had other ideas.

He got off the ship, promptly met another heavy drinker from our ship (Tom) and the two of them headed straight to the nearest island watering hole, where over the course of two hours ashore they sunk 11 cans of very cheap, very heavy island lager, *each*.

Michael somehow made it back to the ship, although he lost all powers of speech for several hours. He was then spotted on the lido deck, unconsciously sunning himself in long black pants, black shirt and lace-up shoes. Perhaps he was in mourning.

And Tom?

Well, nobody ever saw Tom again.

Fast forward a few months, to another cruise tale. I know, it sounds like we're always cruising – but the plain truth is drinkers love cruises, because there's unlimited drinking, and no driving involved. Just bear with me; it all gives further context to the many ways that drinking overtakes one's life.

Anyway, so we're departing Fremantle on the P&O Pacific Jewel's handover to a Singapore purchaser. And as a nod to our noble vessel leaving Australian waters on its final voyage, the staff have lined up literally hundreds and hundreds of *free* yellow and green drinks.

(In actual fact they were green drinks, being Midori and

lemonade, with some fast melting ice in them – but perhaps the staff members pissed in them for the yellow effect). Or maybe the cheap plastic cups were yellow.

Anyway, it didn't matter to me.

Those drinks were sitting out in the sun, waiting for the flag to drop, when people could move in and grab them. So we all hovered about, trying not to look too eager. Because *we* didn't have drinking issues – we could take them or leave them, anytime.

Right?

Well, those drinks sat out in the sun for about an hour. The ice completely melted, the fizz unfizzed, and a lot of the hopefuls had kind of meandered back to the bar, or their sun lounges – when suddenly the whistle went.

I began to move over towards the table, and to my amazement, everyone around me leapt into gear – FREE DRINKS!!! – and they were scooping up five or six of them, saying they were taking them back for friends. Which they might have been.

But I was mortally outraged at this, after having waited so long. And also, I was more scared of missing out! So I muscled Michael up to the drinks table, and we scooped up a handful each.

I started scoffing the revolting warm green liquid down. By now, those drinks looked like plastic cups of Draino. Michael sipped his, didn't like it, and passed it over to me. And I managed to imbibe at least six of them.

I didn't enjoy them, in fact they were revolting. But they were alcohol, and most importantly, they were *free*.

And that, my friend, is how Drinking Brain thinks.

There's no moderating something so mindless.

A quick segue into the eager uptake of drinks packages on cruise ships – aren't they just grand? I had a drinks package on a 14 day cruise once – and all it meant was I needed to drink at least 9 beers a day, every day, in order to break even on the financial outlay of roughly a thousand bucks.

Only diehard drinkers like me would ever think this was good financial management.

#

Anyway, I guess that covers moderation, and the reverse, in action. I just wanted to illustrate how the drinking brain reacts to the idea of light, or mid strength - and especially, free alcohol.

It's the same with wine. I have friends who'd buy low alcohol wine when they went out to, say, a barbecue they had to drive home from. But they never bought the light stuff because they wanted to – it was simply to enhance the chances of getting home without losing their driver's licence. And it didn't even always work out for them!

Whereas what they needed all that time was a vehicle they could sleep in, like my van. Something no dedicated drinker should be without.

Another moderation technique I tried was the two drinks a day agenda. Another cracker of an idea, courtesy of my never-fail Drinking Brain. I figured if I just knew I could have two beers a day, I could be satisfied with that.

It's like being allowed to have two rows of chocolate when you're dieting. Sure it's not as much as you want, but it's a darn sight better than none.

Michael made a rule that you couldn't roll over your drinks to the next day, which peeved me, because I could have saved mine up for a royal weekend binge. But all that rule made me do was ensure I drank two beers a day, every single damn day, just so I wasn't 'missing out.'

Drinking Brain will *not* let you miss out, if it can help it.

So that lasted a while, and then failed, interestingly on a cruise ship again.

Anyway - every moderation idea my drinking brain came up with, Michael would go along with, nodding in his sublime, wise old owl way which I found infuriating. Because he had already tried everything, you see. Over his years of attempting to moderate, or even stop, he had employed every strategy he could think up. And he's got a good brain, so he'd covered off on most things.

He'd even been to an alcohol counsellor, and was about a year into that when I met him.

How was that going for him?

Well, nowhere.

He drank, and saw a counsellor about his drinking. And the counsellor enabled his drinking by suggesting ways to perhaps drink less, but within the limitations of life being stressful, so maybe it's not the right time to 'give up' now, Michael.

Michael agreed with his counsellor, and kept right on drinking.

(Remember the chapter about the system enabling the drinking? There's money to be made out of drinkers – we are the product, not the alcohol. A bit like social media.)

My arrogance and ego stepped in as well, regarding moderation creativity. Every single part of me had a sincere crack at it. I would say, well, I used to land planes as a career, so I can surely find a way to keep drinking!

Such is the desperation - overlaid with superiority, arrogance, but a healthy dose of fear as well. Because – is it possible I actually *can't* moderate my drinking?

What does that then make me?

Problem drinkers can't moderate.

There, I've said it.

Even those who honestly regard themselves as non-problem drinkers - even they, at times, drink more than they intend to.

They lose control.

Such is the nature of indulging in an addictive substance.

They just don't see it as a problem. Just a slip, they say.

And that lack of insight is just part of the overall problem that is alcohol. Because to their minds, the slip has to be either ignored, dismissed – or justified – and none of those options are based in honesty, are they?

The truth is – they lost control.

Why?

Because they're partaking of an addictive substance – and refuse to see what they're doing, and that the substance won that round!

And why do they do that?

Easy.

They want to be able to keep on drinking, because they don't want to live a life free of the stuff. So they turn a blind eye, and tell you they can stop anytime, and it's not a problem.

Yeah, right.

I don't have a lot of time for listening to that sort of crap.

Those people are just as much a problem to themselves, as to admitted problem drinkers like myself. They unwittingly gaslight themselves, and others, out of admitting we as a species are in deep shit around this substance. And there's no hope of finding a solution to a problem that isn't even acknowledged as one.

It's like the lie that is alcohol is all-encompassing, and it's because most drinkers simply want to keep the illusion going.

Because it's easier than addressing it.

Which leaves us with one solution.

One chance.

And that is stopping.

Ending our drinking journey.

Which doesn't mean just stopping drinking. It means looking at ourselves, learning who we are, finding another way to exist.

Day by day.

Until one day, we dismantle that shitty drinking wiring we've carried all through our lives. It falls away – and we are finally free of the scourge.

11

The Decision

So, how do you do it?

Starting at the very beginning – a very fine place to start – (you sang that, didn't you) let's consider where most important life changes occur. And that's with –

THE DECISION.

The decision to no longer drink alcohol needs to occur *in the right time and context*.

This is super important.

Because this kind of decision has to be undertaken when you're actually *not* under the influence of anything. Least of all the alcohol.

You cannot successfully take an important decision like this when you've been drinking, or are in the throes of a hangover (and feeling sorry for yourself) – or when you've got *any* alcohol still in your system.

I'm saying you need to decide, really decide, when you're stone cold sober. When you're at least, say, a week free of the drink.

Why is that?

Because how many times have we all drank to excess, done stupid regrettable shit to people we care about, or have felt like death warmed over, and decided in the moment 'That's IT! No more!'

After all, it's an easy decision you think you're making, while you're remorseful, or while you're physically sick with a thumping hangover. Because it's the *only* logical thing to do.

Right?

Nobody in their right mind would want to keep doing it to themselves.

Of course, it *is* the logical thing to do. But it won't stick.

You're springboarding it straight off the back of a bad reaction.

And as with rushing into an affair with Rebound Guy right after emerging from a dead-end relationship – it's never a good idea – it doesn't last – and you'll feel even worse for having failed yet again.

If you're like most problem drinkers, and like I was, you'll have already made the decision about a hundred times in the past anyway. You might have abstained from drinking for a while – or not – and then fallen back into it. And bashed yourself senseless for failing.

Yes, I know you.

Because as drinkers, even though we may drink for different reasons, and in different styles, the substance itself affects us all pretty much the same way.

We have that commonality of understanding.

So, I'm putting it right here:

The next time you get totally shit-faced, and decide you just cannot keep doing this to yourself – don't make the decision right then and there that you're stopping. Just take a few, sober days to really *feel it*.

Feel the pain.

Feel your thoughts.

Sit sober with those thoughts.

This is the hard part - but it's going to set you up for success.

Feeling is the way through this, and out the other side.

It's sitting with the hard emotions, feeling them, owning them – and then releasing them. And believe me, it is the *only way* out the other side.

Numbing those crap feelings or thoughts with another drink will merely put you back to where you began, and ensure you *never* get off that shitty merry go round.

Pick up a couple of books on the topic of addiction – hell, pick up *this* book – and allow it to sink into your psyche.

While you're sober.

You cannot *feel* unless you're sober.

You don't feel when you're numb.

And you don't feel when you're hungover – except sorry for yourself, and reactive.

And therefore, it follows that you can't feel your way through the problem, and out the other side of it, unless you're clear-minded. And it takes a few days after that last drink for the alcohol to make its way out of your system. So then you can face exactly where you're at, examine what's in front of you, and *decide, really decide*, which way you want your future to look, and be.

This is a great time to revisit that exercise I talked about earlier.

Remember where you made those two lists – one for why you drink, and the other for why you want to stop – and then looking at the conflicts there? Now is the time to dig those babies out, and really, really examine them, with your Beautiful New Clear Head.

Sit down in the sun, with a delicious cuppa, and some lumberjack cake, and really absorb what's going on here. How you were drinking for one reason, but how your drinking seemed to create or further perpetuate that reason to *keep* drinking. And always, *always*, it numbed and delayed your opportunity to ever solve that problem you were drinking for.

You're already halfway there, can you believe it?

Because you're now at the point of being sober (not drink-affected, not full of buyers remorse, not afflicted by hangover) and therefore you can really make a conscious and sober decision about your future!

How bloody exciting is that!!

You now get to *choose* how your life is going to change, to be gloriously different, and never, ever have to deal with the painful conflict that is drinking ever again.

Don't believe me yet?

Keep reading.

#

Armed with your newfound understanding around your drinking, and the realisation that alcohol fixes *absolutely nothing* – try and think of a good and valid reason to drink alcohol. How it actually, genuinely fixes anything for you.

Go on.

I'll wait.

I'll finish my cake.

(It doesn't matter if you can't come up with anything at this point. And if you can – please shoot it through to me on my substack. I welcome all observations from readers.)

#

So having made your decision – and this time it's a clear headed, rational and responsive decision, possibly for the first time ever, now you get to start addressing the pathetic, deceitful lie that is alcohol, and all the pissweak reasons your own drinking brain will fling at you in horror, as it realises you're now armed with a weapon it never knew you had:

Rational Undrinking Strategies – congratulations! - you're now coming from a strengths-based perspective.

Your drinking brain, now encountering the new neural wiring you're beginning to lay the tracks for, will not like it one little bit.

Be warned.

After all, it's used to dealing with, and defeating your willpower. It knows your willpower wears out, because it always has. It just needs to lie in wait, for a difficult day to come along, and then assert itself – and bingo – your drinking brain will be headed to the bar, waving your debit card.

But what's going on *here*?

What, you're actually questioning drinking brain? You're saying that alcohol *isn't* your friend? And worse, why it isn't?

Wait – you *know* this??

Who bloody told you that!? drinking brain screams like a hysterical toddler.

So now you go to work on it, hour by hour, day by day.

This is where the work you do really, really comes into the picture.

You move one stubborn old festy brain-brick at a time, and replace it with a fresh new modern one. Ah, so much lighter.

Some days you might have drinking brain attacking you many times, or almost continuously, depending on how and why you used alcohol in the past - and other days you'll be blissfully free of it. Or it will have a little go, and retreat with barely a whimper.

But be warned, it won't give up easily. And even as time goes on, that little sucker will still give you a less-hopeful nudge, even knowing its chances are miniscule. But it wouldn't be alcohol and addiction if it didn't just keep on trying.

I'll jump in now with what my drinking brain threw at me -

'You can't go for a walk to the beach. You'll see people drinking at that pub you walk past. It'll make you miserable. You'll have to hide at home for the rest of your life – and never go to that beach again.'

(The beach has always been my sanity.)

I can tell you, I *didn't* walk past the pub, my usual route to the beach, that day. I went another way, and thought about how I felt.

And then I *felt* into my feelings, as I walked along, noticing new things, different houses and gardens, and people. I talked to people – and really looked at them.

Because I wasn't sitting in a pub drinking, I had the time to.

And what I was feeling was I'd made the decision, and although it felt strange walking a different way to the beach, I knew I was going to do a *lot* of things differently from here on. And this was in fact a *good thing*!

And I arrived at the beach, plopped myself into that crystal clear water, and felt bloody amazing, for being alive, for *having found a way, today*. And funny, I no longer felt like I'd missed out on anything at all.

When I walked home, it was past that same pub.

No problem.

And the next time I went to the beach, I just walked my usual way.

I'd thought about it briefly, realised I didn't need to fear drinking anymore, so I didn't need to walk a longer distance. I knew I'd be okay in this particular scenario now. And I saw those people drinking. And my drinking brain tried to whisper in my ear that that was what I liked to do, jibing a little memory in there – but I kept right on walking.

Because I remembered how great that sober swim had felt last time, and the power I had basked in that day.

I was unconsciously strengthening the new neural path I'd begun creating for myself, on the back of that memory.

I wanted to do that again, to feel that power, way more than I could imagine wanting that drink!

I had laid down a new neural pathway already. An option, to do something good, something better and powerful for Me. And I was reinforcing that, every single time I choose Me, and my *power*, over a serve of alcohol.

THE DECISION

Now at this point, I want to be clear on what I was *not* doing:

I was not thinking 'I have to *give up* drinking.' Giving up something would have implied I wanted to hang on to it, but was telling myself I couldn't have what I still wanted. And I wasn't telling myself I *can't* have a drink – but rather that I'm *choosing to be free* of the drink. Because the moment your self-talk goes to FOMO – fear of missing out - that's where willpower will be the only resource you have to call on. You're fighting a battle in your own head every single time, by doing it that way. You're feeling a sense of *lack*, when you label what you're doing as "giving up" something.

Why do it the hard way?

Why not call on the infinite resources inside you, that most powerful possession you have – your Brain – and use it, to unconsciously bring about the change you want?

Because your own self-talk is incredibly powerful. You can either choose to train your brain into feeling free of alcohol, or conversely, 'giving up' alcohol. One implies effortless freedom, but the other suggests you miss out on something you still want. And that puts you straight back into that dichotomy of, 'I know it's bad for me, but I still want to do it.'

You want it to be effortless, right?

So your self-talk will be, 'I no longer choose to drink.

No thanks, I'll pass on that whole idea.'

No room for argument.

Think of your drinking brain as this monster toddler inside your head.

If it wants something you don't, you don't reply with, 'I know it's hard, but you're going to have to *give that up.*' Because that leaves the door open for an argument.

Just kick that door shut with a resounding No!

(If you happen to have a toddler, next time you're at the supermarket checkout and they want a Kinder Surprise, reassure them that they'll enjoy being free of those also. And then let me know how it went - I'm really interested!)

Back to you.

What you're aiming at here is your ultimate prize – and that prize is EFFA –

Emotional Freedom From Alcohol.

(Goes well with the FFS, don't you think??)

Emotional freedom from having these battles in your head around drinking.

Freeing up your head space from thoughts of alcohol. No longer wasting neurons on deciding when you'll drink next, and how much, and who with, and what it will cost and can you afford it, and where you can buy it the cheapest in bulk, and how you'll get home after drinking, and how much you can drink and still drive, or what way you'll drive home if you've had too much, or how much will an Uber cost, and should you preload, to make this expensive night a bit cheaper ... All that shit thinking, taking up major hard drive in your brain, that can be filled with gloriously beautiful experiences that don't give alcohol even a megabyte of space in your mind.

Freeing yourself from your mental prison, to let in all the good stuff.

Great experiences, great people, great times. And drive home safely after them, each and every time. And sleep a deep, refreshing sleep, every night, to awake each morning, greeting the new day with a clear head and a hopeful, positive mindset.

(I swear, sometimes birds suddenly appear when I wake up in

my sunny bedroom. Doves. You should see them.)

Sounds like a fairy tale to a drinker – and yet it's really so close.
 Just changing your thinking, one brain wave at a time.
 Challenging the old ways, to usher in the new.

Here's another one of my drinking brain's attempts:
 I'm travelling around country Queensland, and arrive at a beautiful old pub. I'm thinking I'll be sitting on that big old veranda shortly, where there's nothing quite like a parmy – *and a beer* whispers drinking brain.
 I look around, at the beer garden ablaze with bougainvillea, and the palms nodding in the clearest of blue outback skies. And I think, how will drinking alcohol make me *more present* in this amazing place, make me appreciate and enjoy it more than I already am?
 And I know of course it can't – for the simple reason I'll be focusing on the drink in front of me, rather than the splendour all around. Because alcohol takes you *out of* the moment – *not* more deeply into it, as we're led to believe.
 And once I've ordered my parmy, and an iced lime soda to go with it, I sit in that beautiful space, and really, really *notice* what's going on around me – as opposed to embracing a foggy feeling that would start to clutch my brain after the first few gulps of alcohol, as much as my hand would clutch that glass until I'd emptied it.
 I am so enjoying sitting here in this space, no alcohol could make this better.
 And if I don't quite 100% believe it yet, my drinking brain *doesn't know that*!

Drinking brain has rat cunning, but it's pretty damn slow and stupid really.

It's our lowest self.

Drinking brain just observes me rejecting it, yet again, for the real, tangible pleasures of what's already around me. And drinking brain is weakened, each time I choose against it. And I can tell you, it's not too many more times like this that old drinking brain no longer even bothers to pipe up. It knows it's pointless, in this situation anyway. It'll wait for a different scenario.

And I know I have laid down new wiring.

It didn't happen straight away, but with repetition, this one eventually took hold as well, and cut that shitty old programming for good.

Here's another one, a little different – and this one nearly became a slip! But on this day, God stepped in, or the Universe, or whatever you like to call Him. God helps those who help themselves, as my mother used to say...

I'm walking down the main street at lunch time, and I see a sign at the bistro. They've got my favourite pub fodder, rissoles and mash and gravy. I dive in, this time not even really thinking. The wait staff looks at me, and these words pop out of me: 'I'll have the rissoles please – and a Great Northern.'

Yep, old programming.

Sneaky.

As the waitress starts totting it up, my brain is trying to process what just happened.

Did I just order a beer?

I did.

Do I want that beer?

Hmm. Well, I ordered it. Maybe I'll just have it.

Just have a pot, not a schooner, suggests drinking brain helpfully. *I know you want to control your drinking now. A little pot, you won't even feel that...*

'I'm sorry, you'll have to order your drink at the bar in there,' the waitress hooks a thumb towards the dark gaping maw of the public front bar. Okay, I say, and hand over the money for just the rissoles. And I then move towards the bar.

Drinking brain is keeping quiet – and I'm thoughtful. *Don't overdo it*, I can feel drinking brain's line of thought. *You're going in. We're having just one beer today.*

Ah – at last.

I enter the bar, and I look around. I see about six souls in there, each clutching their glass in the darkness, even though it's such a magnificent day outside. They sit in that dark space, alone, brooding, lost in themselves, staring into the (piss) in front of them.

Something in me literally gasps at how easy it is to fall into the trap that is alcohol.

I might add, at this point I had around nine months of sobriety behind me. Yet here it was, so easy, the trap set and ready for me.

Yet, nine months of sobriety now shone a spotlight on what I was looking at here – and it wasn't one bit enticing. In fact, it looked like a dark horror show to me. I saw those sad looking souls, lost to the demon drink. And I saw how easily I'd been led, even duped into perhaps having just one pot.

To rejoin that party from hell.

The barman approached me and asked what'll it be – and my mouth instantly replied 'Coke with ice thanks.' Some of the souls at the bar looked up momentarily, with dead eyes. And then I paid, and was out of there, into the garden area, my soft drink thankfully in hand.

I fully recognised the near miss – and how on this occasion the Universe had stepped in to show me, because I now held my own light and was able to see through the darkness, and choose No.

Because of this, I believe I attracted the help I needed that day.

You will have many, many experiences like these.

I could go on for chapters of examples, but I want to keep this book short and sweet and to the point. Punchy.

Sometimes drinking brain will come at me with clear directions. It will appeal to emotions, to habits, to subconscious wiring. And sometimes it will just fling a drink order into my brain, like it did that day – and then a miracle happened, and I'd had to go indoors into a dingy, smelly bar full of lost souls, to re-order the alcohol – *if I'd really wanted it.*

And I didn't want to, once I saw what was waiting for me, on the other side of that drink.

Yet nine months prior, it would have been automatic – and I can tell you, I wouldn't even have *seen* the sadness in there. I would have seen fellow drinkers, and I likely would have nodded or chatted to them, as I ordered my own poison. I might have even sat in there, in the dark with them, rather than outside in the fresh air. And I know my rissoles wouldn't have tasted anywhere near as good – because I would have been focused on the alcohol – and alcohol dulls all other experiences in its wake.

Nine months ago though, I didn't know any of this. And you

can only work with what you do know.

Reading this book, you, dear reader, will know what I'm talking about. And you'll get to choose all of your experiences. One at a time. Each experience taking you further and further away from the lie that is alcohol, into the light that is presence, and choice.

It's really just a paradigm shift, put simply. Because everyone has a different life perception, or viewpoint – therefore it can be changed, at the will of the person. So essentially the change can only ever happen from your viewpoint, or point of perception. And if you choose to see things differently (alcohol specifically) so you will learn to react to it differently.

Remember, every belief you hold around alcohol came from somewhere. You weren't born with those beliefs. You learnt them, and you then went on to reinforce it, until you no longer even realised you're viewing your need to drink through that lens, which is your own personal Life View.

But once you start challenging those beliefs you hold, and realising they really are just erroneous and very unhelpful wiring, you can then begin the task of sifting through those beliefs, keeping those that are useful to whatever it is you're wanting to change (in this case your reliance on alcohol) and discarding those beliefs which do not serve your shiny new viewpoint.

Replacing those discarded beliefs with new, productive truths will enable the path to lasting change for you, without any willpower having to be spilt in the exercise. You will simply follow your beliefs, as before, but the difference being that these new beliefs will serve your desire to be in your own sober truth, rather than drinking with the same old herd, in the same old way, with your same old problems. Stuck.

It's really that simple.

Because what's really the alternative?

Now you know - alcohol eventually replaces all of your desires to do anything that you once did.

Alcohol is a drug.

It can also be likened to an all conquering monster that has no interest whatsoever in your well being, but disguises the gradual undermining of you by giving highs - but highs which reduce the desire to seek highs and satisfaction from worthwhile pursuits.

It destroys your soul, and the possibilities of your life journey with it.

It's evil - and yet it's a belief you can unlearn.

No more, no less.

Every belief has a counterpoint. So anytime you used to say you were "giving up" drinking (implying loss) and replace it with *freeing yourself* from alcohol (implying freedom) that in and of itself is a huge change in viewpoint.

I choose to be free from alcohol.

I choose *not* to follow the herd.

I choose to be present at all times, for everybody I care about, but especially for myself.

I choose to work on, and solve my problems, so they no longer exist.

I choose to sort my problems out, not numb them.

I choose my own health and wellbeing.

I choose not to be an embarrassing drunk.

THE DECISION

I choose Me, over any type of alcohol in the world.

I choose....
Grace over Ego – in all things.

#

Quick fixes: swapping substances.

A short note on swapping your alcohol addiction for another, because this is more common than I ever would have believed.

I'm noticing people compare weed addiction to alcohol addiction, for instance. Or if you ever go to an AA meeting, you'll notice many participants are nicotine fiends.

I'm sorry, but I'm going to crash the delusion here, to say this does nothing from the perspective of empowering you to make real choices, *good* choices, that ultimately free you from addictions of *all kinds*.

Because once you get into the duality of arguing over which addiction is better or worse – well, sad to say, you're still an addict, and still not steering your own life. The substance is. And whether it's a better one or not, well, that's your own viewpoint yet again, just so you can enable another addiction. One person's dope is another person's heroin is another person's vape is another person's ketamine.

Arguing over what's worse is semantics, and frankly pointless.

The idea here is that if you can subsist in presence through your problems and pain, you'll come out the other side without needing a damn thing to numb it away.

How's that for an idea, life being simple like that!

I'm not saying life is easy, by any stretch.
Sometimes it's bloody hard.
But addictive substances do nothing towards making those times easier, and work against them *ever* improving for you.

Why stay stuck wallowing in your own misery, just so you can numb it for a few hours of the day, but remain trapped in it? Why not just step out of the pile of shit you're in, smell the turds stuck to your boots, but then wash off that mess, and move on with your life? You're not going to step out of a pile of dogshit to then say, hmm, I'll go lie down in this cowpat because it doesn't smell *quite* so bad – are you?

You're reading these words from a person here who initially swapped my alcohol problem for a sugar addiction. Although truthfully, I've been addicted to sugar my whole life. I just didn't really understand it for what it was.

Yep, another addiction!

But the interesting thing about all of this is once you learn that staying trapped in addictive ruts does nothing for you, and that the way to lift yourself out of them is by shifting your beliefs around how the substance serves you – then you can literally step out of *anything!*

It's all done by using the power of the mind that we are all born with, but frequently forget to use.

That power rests with YOU.

12

It's More Fun Not Drinking!

What if you could create a life that good that you didn't have to escape into a bottle in order to keep living it?

Really, really think about that idea.

Do you find it appealing?

Or do you find it difficult to believe that it's even possible?

I'm going to finish this book on a high note, and make good the claim that it's actually *way* more fun not drinking!

Can't imagine it?

Well, here's a few tools to help you visualise it – and not to worry, because soon you'll be doing all of this, firsthand!

Let's start by picking a type of outing you enjoy, and where you usually drink when you do it. In my case, I'll go with running a social event.

I always drank at those times. In fact, I'd preload before I even got to these events, as I felt I wouldn't be funny or interesting enough without the alcohol. So I'd drink before, I'd drink during, and I'd keep drinking until I somehow got home and crashed into bed, on my way to the perfect hangover the next day.

And I somehow believed I was having fun doing this. Over and over again.

One of my favourites was a sunset cruise on the Noosa River.

I'd arrange to meet a group of people there. So, about an hour beforehand, I'd start drinking. And by the time I got there, I'd be somewhat affected.

(Refreshed, I used to call it!)

I'd go there, find my people, and there would be hugs all round, and feigned delight at seeing all of them. Yes, even the ones I couldn't stand. Then it's off to the bar, sooner rather than later, so that the alcohol wouldn't wear off! I'd stand in a queue at the bar.

The boat would depart, and I'm still standing downstairs at the bar, in the bowels of the boat, waiting to be served my alcohol. At last.

We'd be cruising down the river – but I'd forget to enjoy the cruise, because I spent all my time crapping on about nothing, and drinking (I might as well have been sitting in some dingy old bowls club). By the time we'd get to the sunset part of the cruise, I wouldn't even know we'd arrived. If I was lucky though, somebody might announce it, and then I'd leap up so I could drunkenly fire off a heap of sunset snaps through my phone, to post proudly on Facebook – but as for *enjoying* it with any kind of presence – well suffice to say I needed those photos to prove I'd even been there, let alone remembering any of it!

Then it was back to the bar for more drinks on the return trip (which I frequently couldn't remember *anything* of) and then from there I'd kind of ooze across to the worst fish n chippery in town with the others (the sober ones protesting that the food there was pricey and awful, but their protests being shut down by the drunks). And there, after waiting about an hour for a costly piece of parched fish and some oily chips (but still drinking) I'd mindlessly shovel in this garbage, then head over to the RSL club to not hear whatever band was playing.

I might get fondled up by some revolting drunks, and then somehow arrive home in one piece, to collapse onto my bed. It's a bugger I drank so much though, because the surfing I'd planned to do the next morning would have to be cancelled, as I lay groaning on my bed, my head thumping, and feeling queasy and regretful. I'd then lie to my surf buddy about why I couldn't go surfing.

Feeling sick, I'd say.

No, it's not a hangover. Just came on.

Aah, another great night out, I wouldn't think.

But contrast this:

I'm attending the Noosa sunset cruise with a select few friends whom I really like, and who I'm really, really looking forward to catching up with. I get ready - and I'm actually looking organically beautiful in my well-hydrated skin - as I head over to meet them.

I have a pre-cruise icy soda, or maybe a cappuccino – and I'm admiring the beauty of the river at the harbour, and the way the sun reflects off the many colourful boats moored there. Music is playing somewhere.

Soon, we're boarding our boat, and chatting with Chris, the captain – he's a lovely fellow who's captained this glorious old river boat for 30 years. But he's always got new stories to tell.

Once we're on our way, we marvel at the scenery, and the

waterbirds, as well as the crafty falcons fighting for our leftover food.

(Wait – there's actually *food* on this cruise??? In all these years, I never knew that!)

All too soon, we've arrived at sunset point, but way before that we've been soaking in the tranquility, and marvelling at the palette of colours in the slowly darkening sky, which are reflected onto the water in every direction.

I'm so very, very blessed to be here, filled with gratitude in fact, as I look around at the smiling faces of my friends as they too drink it all in. Sometimes we're silent, so mesmerising is the sensory experience on offer.

I take a few photos, but it can't compete with the moment itself.

All too soon, we are turning back to harbour. The wind is a bit chill now, as we huddle into our coats (I remembered mine this time). And when we get back into harbour, we *select* some delicious food from the plenty that's on offer at the marina. In no time, we're sitting down, passing platters, and recapping on what a great evening it's been.

Should we go dancing? Some of us want to, so we find out what bands are playing close by. And if they're good, we might go – but I know I'll remember every aspect of the night, I'll sing along to the good stuff, and dance my little socks off. And no drunks will even think to touch me up - because they'd just be confusing their ambitions with my capabilities to humiliate them by suggesting they fuck off and take it elsewhere. So they'll go hassle someone else.

And when I'm ready to, I'll *choose* to go home at the end of it, tuckered out and happy, but remembering to say goodbye to my friends this time. Best of all, I have the certainty of waking early in the morning for whatever activities I'd planned for the next day.

The same activity – one as an unconscious drinker and one as a conscious undrinker.

(Try saying that one fast, three times).

And ask yourself which one do you prefer the sound of?

Take a moment to visualise your own activities, looking at them through the lens of a drinker. And be real about it. It's easy to think, 'Oh I had a great time Friday night. Yeah, I met up with my mates, we sunk a few, um, then I can't remember that much, but hey we had a great time, and I can't wait to do it again. Except I'm glad it's not right now, because my head's still thumping.'

Really *pull it apart*, and analyse it.

How much of it was truly a positive memory of great fun, where you were actually present for those moments – and how much of it was unconscious belief, or habit?

Then picture it, in your mind's eye, without alcohol present.

Can you even picture it?

Because if you can't, or you're struggling with this concept, it's time to accept that you're *only* there for the alcohol, not the activity itself.

Take it from me, I was a person who thought I was enjoying kayaking in a group, when really it was the six pack I carried in an esky onboard with me. I could never remember much of the actual kayaking event itself!

I think of all the bands I used to go and see on a Friday night – and I know in my heart that if someone had said I couldn't drink at those venues, I likely wouldn't have bothered going.

So what does that tell me?

Now it's your turn.

Have a think about those activities, and then picture not being allowed to drink at them. Would those events, or friends for that matter, hold the same attraction?

It's time to start looking at activities you *genuinely enjoy*, as opposed to activities you partake in purely because there's alcohol involved. It's easy to make that demarcation, by the way.

Genuine activities don't require a mind-altering substance to enjoy the experience. And once you drop the drink, you'll realise there's a whole world of amazing pastimes to get into, that don't involve a drop of alcohol being spilt!

And it's the same with your friends. This is the time you'll really notice who your real friends are. And by the time you come clean of the alcohol, you'll find you've also cleansed yourself of what you thought were friends, even deep and meaningful ones, but which now don't seem to fit in with your new, clean life.

It's not that you can't keep them as friends - but you'll realise you don't really click with those people anymore, *unless there's some authenticity to that friendship.* But you don't even need to know that, or work on it - it will just magically happen.

As you yourself become authentically present, you will find that those who aren't authentically interested in you will just fall by the wayside.

That may sound sad, or scary, or lonely to you now. But it isn't.

New people will come into your new non-drinking life, and they'll be there for You, not because you drink an addictive substance with them. And you'll form real and authentic attachments with these friends, and they to you.

You might even find some of your old friends fall into this basket too. Perhaps they were sitting there all along, waiting for the real You to emerge out of that bottle, so that now they can connect with you in a powerful, authentic way.

This is what happened to me. And it's all fantastic!

Life's too short and beautiful, to waste it being wasted.

#

Drinking doesn't add to your experiences. It subtracts.

Drinking doesn't make you more confident. It's just that once you learn to rely on alcohol for your confidence (faulty neural wiring) - you will then find it impossible to be confident without it.

This is how alcohol works on the brain.

Again, it takes away from you.

It dupes you into believing it's of benefit to you, and that you can't do without it.

But it gives you nothing, except a false belief, that will hook you into coming back for more. Forever - if you don't address it.

It subtracts your options.

It subtracts your memories.

It really, really subtracts the dollars from your wallet, both in the actual drinks ingested at the event, but also in preloading, and by having to pay for Ubers and cabs so you can even get to and from places - and that's not even mentioning your home stock, always at the ready, at the expense of other things you and your family could be enjoying together instead. That thing called quality time.

Drinking subtracts your joy.
It subtracts your presence.
It subtracts your honesty and integrity, and self-worth.
It subtracts your family, and your real friends – the ones you don't have to drink with.

Drinking brain will have you believe that it's more fun when you're drinking.
What it means is drinking brain has more fun – but that's because drinking brain has no discernment, and no presence when it's drinking. And neither do you.
You're just along for the ride, on wherever drinking brain wants to take you. And sometimes, it won't be 'too bad.' And sometimes it's awful, or embarrassing, or downright dangerous or risky.
But is 'not too bad' really as good as you want your life to be?

#

Once drinking brain stops calling the shots in your life, you can fly, baby.
Soar with the eagles, to anywhere, anyhow, with anyone.
You can always hold your own, in any company, and in any conversation.
Being sober in a drinking world is incredibly powerful.
You get to choose how you behave, and who with. Not the drink.

You choose your conversations, and reactions.
You get to keep your memories, all of them, good and bad.
You get to look out for yourself, and your family and friends.
And you get to choose your next direction, every time.

Your confidence will be authentically coming from You - not from a bottle.

And yes, it takes time.

You've had a lifetime of faulty wiring, so it's going to take a little while to unpick that snarl in your psyche. But as you patiently work your way through your rewiring process, your joy (and self-esteem especially) will increase exponentially when you realise you need alcohol for absolutely nothing - and that all that shit did was hold you back from being your Best and Most Glorious Authentic Self.

As a drinker, I'd need at least four drinks before I'd get up and scream out some karaoke - and sometimes even four didn't feel like it was enough - but all I was doing was numbing myself to the whole experience, in case people thought I couldn't sing.

It certainly didn't make me sing better - it just killed off the care factor, and made me sound as melodious as a hooded seal's mating call.

(You can google that one - it involves the seal blowing one of its lungs out of its nostrils, and making a trumpeting phhhfffff noise, causing its eyes to sometimes bleed from the effort. And sometimes the seal doesn't even get lucky. Don't try it.)

Once you lose the Lie that is Alcohol, everything you do becomes authentic - you are now coming from your Self.

And our Selves are so damn amazing!

We're not boring, or lightweight, or any of those labels drinkers use so that they can keep drinking.

We're ourselves.

We're what we were *born* to be, before we became indoctrinated into the lie.

The world just opens up to you in its infinite possibilities, because now you're no longer afraid to be You!

You get to chase your dreams!

What have you always wanted to do, but have felt was 'beyond you?'

For me, it was writing, finishing, editing, and publishing a book. I'd been wanting to do that since I was in high school, over 40 years ago! I have numerous incomplete manuscripts I've started over the decades. Some of them are even good. But I never had the courage, or the focus, to complete what I'd started. Or the time.

Drinking took up so much of my time, and headspace – and health.

But I have the time now. And the focus, and the courage. I might yet become the prolific author I'd always felt I was born to be.

It's ironic that this first book is about alcohol, the thing that has held me back for most of my life. And yet it's just as it should be – because I know this book has the potential to help somebody else overcome the same beast, and step into their future in a completely new and exciting way.

Think of all the possibilities you'll have, with the time and focus and clear head, to steer your own ship at last!

It's never too late to be the inherently glorious creature you were born to be.

And if drinking feels like it's ruling your life – remember that rules are made *by* the broken, *to* be broken.

If you intuitively know that your drinking is harming you, know that your intuition has your welfare at heart.

Always listen to it.

Let it fly!

I wish you all the best on your journey to The Other Side.

13

Q & A Time!

As a bonus...

I thought just for a bit of fun, and further insight, I'd throw this part open to questions from those who've followed my journey thus far. (Some names have been withheld, by request).

The questions relate to anything around the topic of drinking, some of which might not have been covered in this book. And if you, my reader, have any questions you think I may not have answered for you, please send them through to me at cazhow.substack.com – and enjoy a free subscription to my writing while you're there – and I'll get back to you as soon as I can.

I welcome all related questions, and I'm super grateful for your interaction and interest. There are no wrong questions.

These are my own insights, in reply here. It's probably timely now to insert my firsthand experience of problematic drinking, and my observations on life as an Undrinker, as being my qualifications – but that it doesn't make me in any way an "expert" except on my own life experiences.

Having said that, there is no book learning in the world that can compete with real-life experience and struggle, in my view. And if this book goes any way toward alleviating your own curiosity, or is of help to you in your quest towards sobriety, then my mission in writing it is gloriously accomplished!

Enjoy the journey.

#

Random Questions – in no particular order!

Q. What will I do with my time in the evenings if I'm not drinking? I've drank every evening for the last 20 years! PS. I live alone. Thanks, Pamela.

A. Hi Pamela. Thanks for the question. You don't say whether you work during the day, but I'm guessing you fill your day with something other than drinking! So... when you get home, it's likely an opportunity to shift gears for you – and to do the opposite of what your day entailed. After you've nourished yourself with a lovely dinner, perhaps it's a time to brainstorm the things that you would have time for in the evenings, if drinking wasn't taking up all that time. Reading good books and catching a movie always spring to mind, but I'm thinking perhaps it'll be more rewarding to really explore the things in life you've always *wanted* to do, but haven't for whatever reason – and then figure out how to make it happen! Maybe explore some mind maps – they always seem to show up new interesting ideas for me, worthy of further investigation! The rewards will be such that you won't even want to think of drinking as your time-killer anymore. Remember, time is something we all only have a finite amount of. Don't waste it. Good luck.

Q. I have tried to quit so many times, and each time I last about a month, and then have another bender. How do I do this?

A. By turning inwards to understand your unconscious beliefs around alcohol – because that's what's keeping you stuck. Your belief that alcohol 'helps' in some way is what gets you started drinking – and then of course the booze is in control. It's not your friend. It's nobody's friend, despite the way it's glamourised, and universally accepted. It's just an addictive drug, in pretty wrapping, sold in nicely-lit, legal hypermarts, to the masses. Make it your mission to really understand what you're dealing with.Then you can choose to walk away as a free person. All the best to you.

Q. Will I be boring without alcohol, as I'm a shy person?

A. I'll tell you what's boring. Drunks are boring. Except to other drunks. You see, drinking doesn't actually make you more interesting, or fun (although I used to believe that it did). All it does is take away the care factor, so that you no longer *care* if you're boring. And to sober people, Drunk You is probably boring - whereas Sober You would be present, and interesting – and refreshingly different! Does that make sense? Don't worry about being boring as a sober person. The fact you're even questioning it means you definitely *aren't* boring. Good luck!

Q & A TIME!

Q. I'm single, and I go to clubs with friends, meet guys and stuff. But I can't imagine doing this sober? Everyone drinks at these places – amongst other things!

A. Good question. I can tell you, I spent many years going to those places, hoping to meet the right person. But - Drinking Me never ever selected a partner that Sober Me could go forward with for any length of time! Truly, I feel that in these places where, as you say, everyone is drinking, your odds of meeting the right person under those conditions are very, very slim. Have you thought about joining a club or group that does things you're wildly interested in – thereby already having common ground with maybe a future partner? Because when the only common ground is drinking, it's not much to build upon, except more problems down the track. Hope this helps!

Q. Please help. I don't even know who I am without alcohol! I know that sounds pathetic, but it's true. How do I find myself in all of this? - Jenna.

A. Hi Jenna, thanks for the question. I didn't know who I was either, and I really can't say I even cared for a long time, as a drinker. I guess that's called survival mode. You sound like you want so much more than that – which means you'll find it. I know for me it was finally being present with myself, being able to hold bad feelings, and know it wouldn't kill me to do that – and then moving through those feelings by sitting with them, until I found solutions. By doing that, I began building confidence in my Self, and that confidence also served me well in choosing how I wanted to live my life, and starting to choose who my friends were, rather than just letting life happen *to* me.

I could write pages about this – but in essence it's in taking the time to sit with yourself, with a clear, open mind, and finding the peace and grace to keep doing it. And over time, all will be revealed. Hope this helps! Caz.

Q. Okay, this is a bit icky and personal – BUT how do you have sex without drinking? And I'll be anonymous for this one, thank you.

A. I could be a smartass and say 'on my back' but I'm guessing that's not helpful! Um – okay – that's one I'm still figuring out! I have a theory, and that is that without alcohol, I reckon at least 80% of all sexual relations – at the risk of going all Bill Clinton on you –wouldn't ever happen! I could be wrong of course. But I know for me, my sexual journey was very bound up with drinking – and as I'm still working on this one, I'll have to take the question on notice. Just as an aside, a wise old man (my partner's father, actually) once said that 'Sex is an overrated pastime.' Maybe he was right! Though I'm sure Bill Clinton wouldn't have agreed. Thank you. Please feel free to subscribe at cazhow.substack.com (you just need to provide an email address) and reach out further to me at a later date!

Q. Hi Caz. Just about all my friends drink – and I'm really scared if I stopped drinking, I'd be a social leper! What's your thoughts on this? Tayla.

A. Hi Tayla, thanks for your question. I guess it depends on what common ground you have with these friends, outside of drinking events. Do you do things with them that don't involve drinking, such as coffees, or movies, or walks? If you do, then perhaps focus on those people as the friends you have real commonality with, and those activities a bit more. And when you go out to bars, I can tell you firsthand that nobody really cares what you're drinking. It's our own awkwardness around our own non-drinking that creates that divide! If you're confident in choosing not to drink, and being in your truth, nobody will question it, if they even notice it at all! Because getting plastered is really a totally self-centred activity! The problem though is *you* might find yourself getting bored around *them* at those places. Are you ready for that, do you think? Best wishes, Caz.

Q. Hi Caz. You seem on a real downer around drinking. I just wanted to be a bit different here, and remind you that it is legal, not like some other things people do for fun- and if it really was harmful, I'm sure it would be illegal. Everyone needs a bit of fun, right?

A. Unfortunately, being part of a huge drinking cohort is what *doesn't* make you different. I'm sure you also realise there's lots of other substances that are legal too, that are incredibly harmful (cigarettes, vapes, amongst others). As to the 'fun' of drinking – just ask those poor people who end up as victims of violent crime, suicide and the like. Nothing fun there. The fact that something is legal doesn't make it safe, good, or healthy. It just means our governments treat the risk to you as being acceptable – to them.. But how do you feel about those risks, yourself?

Q. Hi Caz. Are you one of those sad AA types, or those weirdos that don't drink - LOL?

A. Hi, Whoever You Are – thanks for offering those labels – but I'm neither. I tried AA and it didn't work for me (too sad I guess) and as for weird, well, that would be correct, in a world where if you don't drink an intoxicating, addictive substance you're deemed weird. I'll take that any day over being the dim-witted drunk that I was. Plus, as a drunk I'd never have attempted to write this book, and you wouldn't have got the chance to ask such a poignant question, right? If you're interested in further discovery of my upcoming and ongoing weirdness, please grab yourself a copy of my book, out soon.

Q. Hi Caz. I'm interested in your book. I've used wine to unwind every night forever, and it's the only thing that helps me cope, and then sleep at night. And I look forward to drinking every night, because I actually enjoy it. What's really wrong with that? Thanks, Marianne.

A. Hi Marianne, thanks for your question. Well, I guess you're the only person who knows if that's your truth, and perhaps you won't really know until you try something different. You say you've done this 'forever.' So... what if you didn't do this? What would you do with yourself each night? Does that frighten you? Is it out of your comfort zone, to sit in sobriety, in full presence with yourself? These are the questions, really. Also, alcohol doesn't actually help anyone 'cope' with anything. It numbs you to whatever problems you have, and so you call it coping with them – but the problems don't go away, because they're never addressed – which gives you an excuse to keep drinking to cope with them. See the trap? I guess the thing to ask yourself is are you happy with your life – and you're the sole judge of that. I know drinking didn't make me happy, or solve my problems. But sobriety does. And that's why I'm sharing the message. I truly wish you all the best.

Q. Someone once said to me that alcohol makes you feel the way you should be able to feel without alcohol. Is this true?

A. Ah, I've heard that one too (and believed it for a long time!) I guess when you look at the effects of alcohol, it enables you to 'feel' less. Less pain, less angst, less everything really. And in place of it, we think we're feeling a high. So, win/win, right? Except it's not strictly true. The 'high' is temporary, it's a chemical reaction to damage occurring to your brain - and it's also the numbing of the Self against its stressors – and in this world we live in where we want the quick fix, it's a pretense that works for a little while. So, I'm thinking we should be able to feel happy and outgoing and unworried without alcohol, for this saying to be valid. And since I stopped drinking, I've somehow become those things without alcohol! It's taken quite a bit of time, I might add. But there you go. Do you want to have to keep drinking to feel that way – or just arrive there organically? It's up to you!

Q. Hi Caz. I know alcohol is bad news, and I've tried to stop drinking so many times. And I really want to! So why do I always fail! What's wrong with me?

A. Hi there, thanks for the question. It's a common story, so please don't feel alone in that. Also, it's an addictive substance, so wondering why it's not easy to break free of it, well, it's no different to wondering why heroin addicts keep going back to their poison also. Because it's *designed* to addict. You don't say what methods you've tried, but I'm guessing a lot of it is relying on willpower – and when you read my book, you'll realise why I believe willpower doesn't work in the long run. Please reach out to me on cazhow.substack.com – I'd be happy to send you a free copy of the book, and really hope it gives you some ideas you mightn't have tried, or some different insights. Best wishes.

Q. Hi Caz. I'm planning on going dry, but my therapist, who I've been seeing a year now, tells me I will fail if I try at the moment, as I have too much stress in my life. Do you think he's right, or is that just an excuse I needed to keep going. Any help appreciated. Lara.

A. Hi Lara. Thanks for your question. I have a friend who went to an alcohol counsellor for a long while too, and received the same advice. In the end, they're in a business, same as everyone else, and I know this sounds harsh, but there's no income for them if you don't drink. You cease to be a customer! In any case, waiting for stress to depart our lives before we can stop drinking is like waiting for hell to freeze over so you can enjoy ice cream once more. Stress is part of life. The trick is being present for it, and feeling your way through it, and solving it, rather than numbing it, which gets you nowhere. Please take a look at my book, I really hope it helps. Kind regards, Caz.

Q. My partner drinks a lot, and we always fight at these times. Will this stop if he stops drinking?

A. It will certainly *change* if he stops drinking. Beyond that, I can't really say, on the amount of detail you give. But you can only work on yourself, and his journey is his own. I hope he stops drinking, so you can start from that point in a more hopeful way. Otherwise, it's like trying to make a relationship work where there's a third wheel involved, that being the drink. And that's who he will turn to, when the going gets tough, not you. It's hard to move forward in that scenario. Regards, Caz.

Q. Why was alcohol an essential service during lockdowns?

A. Well... because apparently that pesky virus couldn't find its way into Liquorland and the like, so it was deemed *safe* to keep drinking. Well, safe for the governments, I mean. Desirable, even. Why? Because it kept you numb, uncombative, unquestioning, and it's how governments control the masses. Check out what happened in Russia years ago, where a pint of vodka was cheaper than a loaf of bread. Drinking was more important than eating bread - unless it's Marie-Antoinette calling the shots; because she preferred you to eat cake! Anyway, it didn't end well for her either.

Q. Do alcoholics ever accept the responsibility for the ripple effects their behaviour creates in the lives of others, i.e. an alcoholic mother's neglect of her only daughter?

A. If you're referring to an active alcoholic, I'd say no. Alcoholism is a disease of denial – but that doesn't necessarily mean the drinker doesn't have awareness of what they've created; it just means they will keep drinking more, as it's too painful to face. Facing up takes courage – and people often drink to escape that exact reality. It's incredibly difficult for those raised by alcoholics. I am one of them, and I too didn't want children as a result. I had awareness around alcohol as a terrible thing, yet I still fell into problem drinking as an adult, due I suspect to childhood traumas... I strived to be the mother I never had growing up, and looking back now, I can see clearly the two conflicting parenting styles I engaged in, as a drinker and as a non-drinker. Thankfully, I have a very close relationship with my daughter, but it's been built on raw honesty, and trust – admitting all my failings, with no excuses – and not sitting in a victim mentality of what my parents did to me, but instead integrating my childhood into my life experience. Because I came to realise that blaming my parents for what I went through, rightly or wrongly, just kept me stuck in powerlessness to change my outcomes. But to reach this understanding takes time, and a willingness to do so. It takes guts to face what pain we cause as drinkers – but it also takes guts for those who've been wronged to step into their own power, and realise they needn't define themselves by bad parenting. They just have to find a new way forward. Shine the light, and all that good stuff.

Q. How many times, if any, have you attempted to quit prior to now?

A. Unfortunately, too many! Those attempts always began during a hangover, and my weapons were logic, common sense and willpower. I found though, that as long as something deep inside me still believed there was some kind of benefit for me in drinking, whether it was confidence or 'fun' or relief or reward – I would always be battling the problem with willpower – and the day would come when I'd fail, once again. You need to go deeper than willpower, to make it stick.

Q. Why is this time "different"?

A. This time began differently for me, because I made the decision to stop drinking forever, around a week after I stopped physically drinking. So there was no pressure on me to make that decision – it came from a place of desiring the outcome, not reacting to the last problem that drinking had caused me. And from there, it was learning everything I could about the psychology of drinking, and beliefs, and how by changing my beliefs, one at a time, and working on them consistently, I really could move mountains. And without willpower.

Q. Do you believe in the concept of having to hit rock bottom?

A. As a drinker, I used to believe that – but I can now see that that belief didn't serve me. It merely gave me the excuse to keep on drinking, by believing, well, I mustn't have hit rock bottom yet! I'm not dead yet! People even used to say to me that once I hit rock bottom, I'd stop. But most weekends felt like rock bottom to me already. I felt bad enough to die, sometimes. How bad does rock bottom have to be, for me to stop? I think 'rock bottom' is just another hurdle to making change; it's like you're waiting for the flag to drop before you do something about it. So, no, I don't believe it's a prerequisite to change. You can make change the moment you make the decision.

Q. Do you believe you could ever become a moderate drinker?

A. As a problem drinker – it's a big No from me. From where I sit now, yes, I possibly could, and I say that because the idea now holds no appeal whatsoever to me. I physically don't *want* to ingest alcohol anymore. But I think when you're in the grip of any addiction, trying to moderate an addictive substance is impossible, both from a physical viewpoint, but especially from a psychological perspective. It just keeps the cognitive dissonance going, and the self-hate when you fail to moderate an addictive substance. Why put yourself through that, all to ingest something that's of toxic harm to your body, your mind and your spirit?

Q. What is your response when people say "Can't you have just one?"

A. While I was still in the mental rewiring stage, and out socially, I was always careful to use explanations such as "I don't drink anymore" as opposed to "I can't drink anymore.' I would tell people, truthfully, I've drank enough alcohol for five lifetimes, and I now choose not to do that to myself anymore! Or I would reply 'I can. I just *don't want to*!' 'I don't need to drink to be here' is another good one. And the best part is these are all responses which bolster the rewiring of one's own beliefs - say it often enough, and in no time you'll really believe it on a subconscious level. It's a bit like meditation. But nobody asks me this question anymore – and I don't expect to be asked it either! Perhaps I just don't put that vibe out there now, and what a relief.

Also - I think "can't" is just one letter away from "can" – and if I was to go around telling my drinking buddies I can't drink anymore – they'd make it their mission to show me I can!

As a dear friend once said to me, 'I can't drink any more,' and upon my questioning it, he quickly replied, 'I can't drink any less either!'

14

Conclusion

Everything is hard before it is easy. – Goethe

Afterword

Please kindly leave a review on this book's Amazon listing, if you found this little book helpful.

Without your valuable review, this book will disappear pretty quickly from Amazon searches - and it can't help others that way. I super appreciate your efforts with this!

(If you're reading this via e-book, just click the Amazon link on the last page.)

Lastly, I'd love to welcome you to a free subscription at cazhow.substack.com - where you can follow my writing, or contact me. (Link on last page also).

I'd love to hear how you're going!

Many thanks.

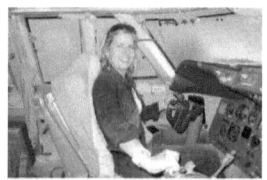

About the Author

Caz How knew she was born to write when her first horror piece disturbed a friend so much that they ended up smashing through their bedroom window, during a nightmare brought on by the story. So, thoughtfully putting fiction-writing on hold (for now) she has instead recorded her own self-help styled memoir of the horror that is addictive drinking.

Decades of drinking had left no time to indulge her passion for writing - so it's ironic that The Social Substance is her first published work, born of four glorious years of mostly effortless sobriety. With a light-hearted tone on what is a deadly serious topic, she manages to instill a well-crafted balance of truth and humor. As she says, if you didn't laugh, you'd cry.

The purpose of this book was always to shine a fearless light on the lie that is alcohol – and most importantly for her readers, show the way out!

These days, Caz spends her time breathing life and colour back into the 90 year old cottage she shares with her partner, Michael, and Aussie Shepherd, Baxter. And in between enjoying mango mocktails from her own garden, she's naturally planning her next book!

You can connect with me on:
🌐 https://cazhow.substack.com

www.ingramcontent.com/pod-product-compliance
Lightning Source LLC
Chambersburg PA
CBHW031251290426
44109CB00012B/533